Surviving and Thriving at Altitude

CHRISTINE EBERT-SANTOS, MD, MPS
ROBERTO SANTOS

Printed in the United States of America
First Printing, 2026

ISBN-13 (Hardcover): 979-8-9941316-0-2
ISBN-13 (Trade Paperback): 979-8-9941316-1-9
ISBN-13 (eBook): 979-8-9941316-2-6

Cover photo by Chris Erickson
Instagram: @ckhock

Isa Publishing
highaltitudehealth.com

TABLE OF CONTENTS

INTRODUCTION

Since 2000 I have been a practicing physician in a small mountain town at 9,000 feet (2,700 meters) elevation in the Colorado Rocky Mountains. I commonly see children with oxygen levels far below normal walking into my clinic showing no trouble breathing. Children with oxygen saturations this low should be very sick. In fact, they should be in the intensive care unit. Parents are told their child has pneumonia or asthma. They are prescribed antibiotics and steroids, even by lung specialists in Denver far below us at 5,280 feet (1,609 meters). These doctors are not seeing what I see.

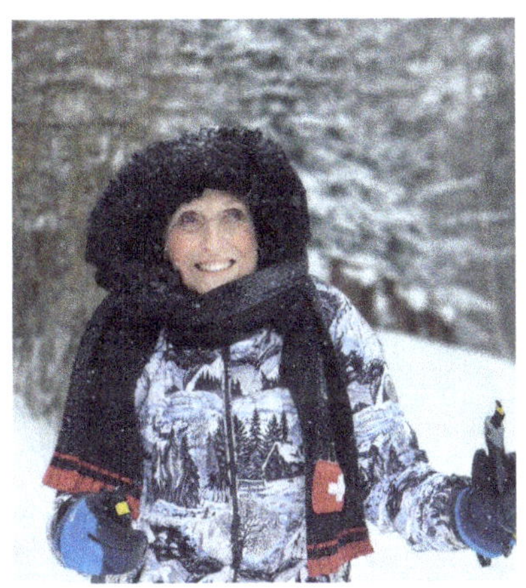

Dr. Christine Ebert-Santos.

Before I opened Ebert Family Clinic in Frisco, Colorado, I spent twenty years working at a hospital in the Northern Mariana Islands, in the remote Pacific Ocean, where the nearest referral center was 3,500 miles (5,600 kilometers) away. I treated severe pneumonia, asthma, tuberculosis, tracheitis, and other complex respiratory conditions. What I see in my high-altitude clinic is different. These children with low oxygen have a previously unrecognized form of **high-altitude pulmonary edema (HAPE)**, now called **high-altitude resident pulmonary edema**, or **HARPE**.

Left untreated this condition can be fatal. Fortunately the remedy is simple: give the patient more oxygen either by means of a nasal cannula or by traveling to a lower elevation.

Outside of the classic scenario where a patient visits from a lower altitude, there is little research being conducted on HAPE and the effects of altitude on mountain residents in North America.

Analyzing data and publishing in scientific journals can take years, even decades, making it difficult for scientists and doctors to share their groundbreaking ideas. Access to peer-reviewed research is very limited and expensive due to this time-consuming process and the exclusive scientific community in which this research is conducted. This is what led to the founding of our blog, highaltitudehealth.com, in 2014.

The blog allows me to quickly post my observations and share the trends in high-altitude research that I learn from conferences and journals. My students, colleagues in high-altitude medicine and science, and children have watched this process and supported it with their own expertise, contributing to a unique body of knowledge that benefits both residents and visitors in our mountain communities.

Previously, there was no other outlet to disseminate information and test new concepts. It is my hope that our blog—and now this book —will give more people access to research and the lived experience of experts, allowing anyone feeling the effects of high altitude to improve their everyday life in the mountains.

The blog gives us an easier and faster way to contribute to medical science. At highaltitudehealth.com, you'll read about The Frisco Score to differentiate HAPE from pneumonia and other clinical discoveries we are developing for peer-reviewed publications. Other topics may inspire scientists and clinicians with more resources and expertise to build on the knowledge we already have.

There are interviews with a cardiologist about the heart, a family practitioner with over forty years' experience, an emergency medical technician and ski patroller, an emergency department doctor, and naturopathic physicians, all sharing their expertise about health at high altitudes. There are articles on the effects on Parkinson's disease, respiratory syncytial virus infections, strokes, kidneys, diabetes, sickle cell disease, ileus, and ticks. Other blog entries describe mountain adventures and misadventures (and how to avoid them) as well as how athletes prepare for competition in a low-oxygen environment. Scientific material includes genetics, physics, the Nobel Prize for studies on hypoxia, research on other mountain populations similar to ours in Colorado (Kyrgyzstan, Peru, and China), and my own research on HAPE, sleep, gout, growth, and other topics.

It is from the blog that the idea for this book was born. We included the material we found most interesting and beneficial, but I encourage you to go to highaltitudehealth.com to find out more, view charts and graphs, and see new articles. We have also included accounts of back-country trips to remote mountain cabins sitting at even higher elevations than those of our tiny mountain towns in Colorado. These excursions are valuable opportunities to observe the body working actively to accommodate the increased demands of decreasing oxygen. That's why I call this book *Surviving and Thriving at Altitude*.

I share my observations in presentations and posters in the community; at scientific conferences; and in newspaper articles, podcasts, and interviews all over the world. Everything I speak and write about is based on patterns seen during decades of clinical observation and data I've collected in my own primary care practice–turned–high-altitude healthcare clinic.

This research continues. I attend in-person and online conferences where scientists share information about the effects of a low-oxygen condition called **hypoxia**. I collaborate with researchers and healthcare providers in communities that have been inhabited by indigenous peoples who have developed unique adaptations to their extreme environments over thousands of years. I also exchange observations with professionals in communities of settlers who have had far less time for their bodies to acclimatize. We are constantly finding similarities and differences between these two different population groups and how hypoxia affects the body.

Meanwhile, with the help of my students, staff, colleagues, family, and everyone who agreed to share their experiences in interviews, I offer you this: twenty-five years of observations at 9,000 feet (2,700 meters) and above.

Christine Ebert-Santos, MD, MPS
highaltitudehealth.com

PART I
WHAT IS HAPE?

The Many Varieties of High-Altitude Pulmonary Edema (HAPE)

High-altitude pulmonary edema, or **HAPE**, can rapidly progress to respiratory failure and death if not recognized and treated. This is particularly dangerous for residents and healthcare providers in mountain communities, who may mistakenly believe they are acclimatized and not at risk for HAPE.

Low oxygen can be caused by being at altitude and by inflammation, which itself is commonly caused by viral infections, such as colds or influenza, but can occasionally occur with bacterial infections, such as strep throat or pneumonia. Low oxygen, or hypoxia, is the result of pulmonary edema, which is when fluid collects in the air sacs of the lungs.

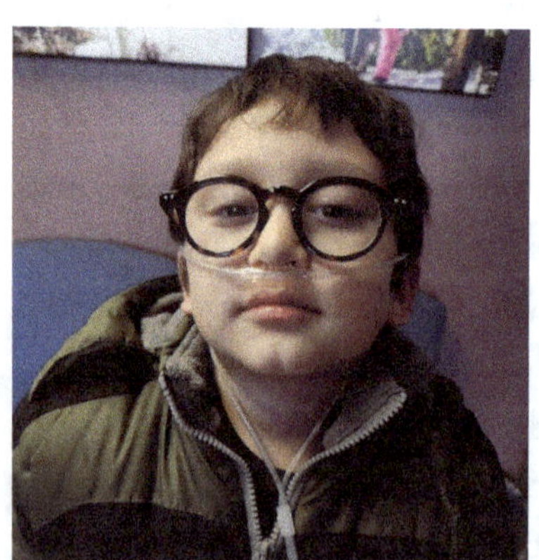

Pediatric patient on oxygen.

There are four types of HAPE:

Classic HAPE has been recognized for over a century. It occurs in visitors to altitudes above 8,000 feet (2,500 meters) beginning within forty-eight hours of arrival. Symptoms include cough, congestion, trouble breathing, and fatigue, which worsen with activity.

Re-entry HAPE occurs in people who live at altitude, travel to a lower altitude, then return home. Symptoms develop within forty-eight hours of returning.

High-altitude resident pulmonary edema, or HARPE, is a recently recognized condition that occurs mostly in children who have an underlying respiratory illness and live at altitude, with no recent history of travel. They have oxygen levels at 89% or lower but do not appear toxic. They are fatigued but rarely have increased work of breathing.

Highlander HAPE occurs when people who live permanently above 8,000 feet (2,500 meters) develop HAPE while traveling to even higher altitudes.

All four types of HAPE can reoccur, but typically not with every arrival at altitude or viral illness.

There is no blood test for HAPE. A chest X-ray may show typical infiltrates seen with pulmonary edema. In mild or early cases it can look normal. Patients with HAPE may also show signs of asthma or pneumonia, which are treated with bronchodilators and antibiotics. Most people with pneumonia at altitude do not have hypoxia or need oxygen, yet many of those who do develop hypoxia are told again and again they only have severe asthma or pneumonia. As a result, they are treated with inhalers and steroids, which usually add nothing to their recovery.

The treatment for HAPE is oxygen, which should be used continuously at a rate that raises oxygen above 90% saturation. The length of treatment may be as short as two days or as long as ten.

If you're at altitude and experiencing a cough, congestion, fatigue, and trouble breathing, use a pulse oximeter to monitor your oxygen levels. This is the best way to keep yourself out of the ER or ICU.

Even Going Back Home to the Mountains Can Be Dangerous

After spending Thanksgiving Day with family in Vermont, **Louie** was excited to hit the slopes the next morning after his return to Colorado. But that night, he noticed he was breathing harder and felt more tired than usual. As a competitive skier Louie thought that was strange. He was still getting over a cold, so he went home early to rest, hoping a good night's sleep was all he needed. He could not have imagined that in twenty-four hours he'd be in the emergency room fighting for his life.

Louie had developed **re-entry HAPE**, a dangerous condition that caused his lungs to fill with fluid, set off by being at altitude and by inflammation from his "cold." His oxygen saturation was 54% instead of the normal 92%. He was vomiting and feeling weak and short of breath. His blood tests showed dehydration, hypoxemia, and acute kidney injury. His chest X-ray looked like a snowstorm.

Louie was transferred to Children's Hospital in Denver and admitted to the intensive care unit. There, the diagnosis of re-entry HAPE was confirmed by echocardiogram, which showed increased pressure in his lungs. With the lower altitude and oxygen treatment, he improved rapidly.

Every year, re-entry HAPE affects several Summit County children, usually between the ages of four and fifteen. Medical providers may not be aware of this risk, assuming children living at altitude are already acclimatized.[1] Inflammation, such as a viral respiratory infection, contributes to the risk. Trauma may also predispose a returning resident to re-entry HAPE.[2]

Most children do not require medical attention after their first episodes. Parents obtain oxygen concentrators for home use when they return from travel and carefully monitor their children's oxygen levels.

Louie agreed to share his story with us to help educate medical personnel and families living in the mountains about this dangerous condition. Further research will help more precisely define who is at risk.

1. See our blog post from April 17, 2019, "Acclimatization vs. Adaptation."

2. As described in our blog post from February 5, 2018, "Trauma Related High-Altitude Pulmonary Edema."

Mountain Residents Can Still Get Mountain Sickness

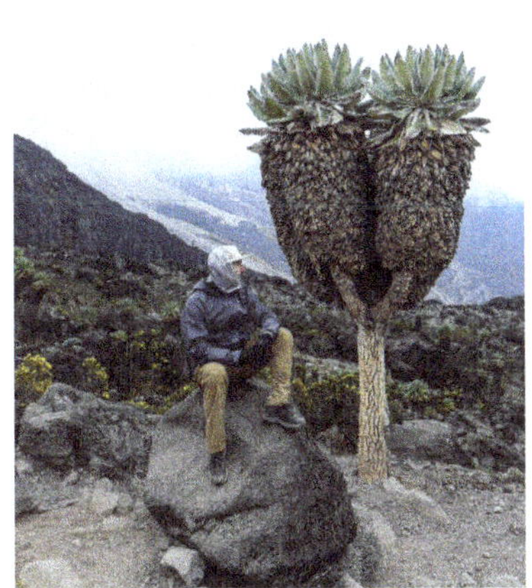

Summit County resident Jonathan Huffman next to a Dendrosenecio kilimanjari, unique to the slopes of Mt. Kilimanjaro.

There are three types of **high-altitude pulmonary edema (HAPE)** recognized in visitors and people living at high altitudes. These include **classic HAPE (C-HAPE)**, which affects individuals who live at low altitudes and travel to high altitudes. **Re-entry HAPE (RE-HAPE)** is seen in people who live at high altitudes, travel to lower altitudes, then return. **High-altitude resident pulmonary edema (HARPE)** occurs in patients who live at high altitude and do not change altitude.[1]

While these have been extensively studied and are subtypes that people are warned of, a fourth, unexpected type of HAPE has been recently described by pediatric pulmonologist Santiago Ucros in Bogota, Colombia, at the Universidad de los Andes.[2]

Highlander HAPE (HL-HAPE) occurs in people who live at high altitudes, then travel to even higher altitudes. Though most people who live at elevation for long periods of time assume they are immune to HAPE, the recognition of HL-HAPE shows this is not the case.

Thirty-seven-year-old **Jonathan Huffman** experienced this when he set out to climb Mt. Kilimanjaro with his wife, Katie.

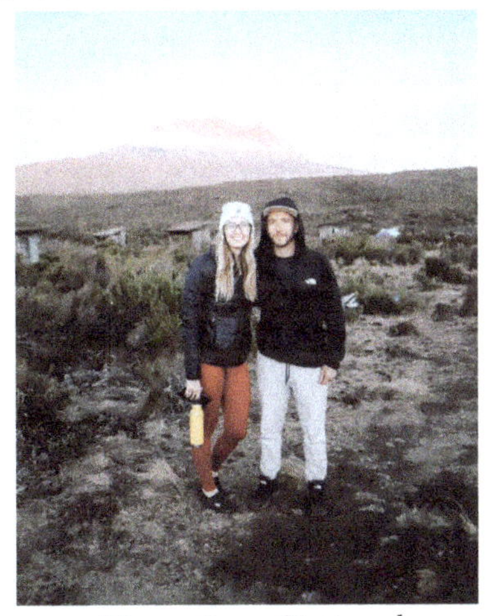

Mountaineers Katie and Jonathan Huffman.

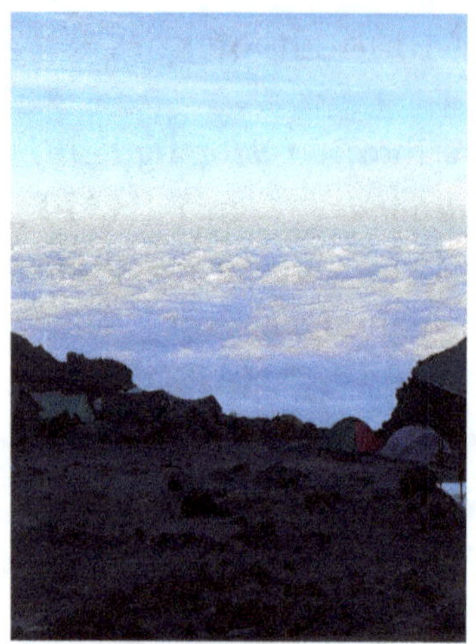

Camp above the clouds on Kilimanjaro.

Originally from Texas, Jonathan had been living in Breckenridge, Colorado, at 9,600 feet (2,900 meters), for fifteen years. In preparation for the climb, he spent the summer hiking multiple fourteen thousand–foot peaks in Colorado, mountain biking, and trail running at 9,000–12,000 feet (2,700–3,700 meters).

Finally, in September, Jonathan and Katie embarked on their long-awaited trip. Upon arrival in Tanzania, they spent two days adjusting to jet lag and preparing for their climb.

The elevation of Mt. Kilimanjaro is 19,341 feet (5,895 meters), and it generally takes each group five to nine days to reach the summit, depending on the route taken. Jonathan and Katie had chosen to follow the Lemosho route, forty-two miles long with an elevation gain of 16,000–17,000 feet (4,900–5,200 meters).

On the first day, when Jonathan and his party started at the Lemosho trailhead (elevation 7,700 feet, or 2,400 meters) and hiked up almost 9,500 feet (2,900 meters) to the first camp, he noticed his throat felt dry and he had to keep clearing it. However, he attributed this symptom to the dusty environment.

The second day was not much better. Jonathan felt as though his body was fighting the dust, which had found its way into his eyes, sinuses, and throat.

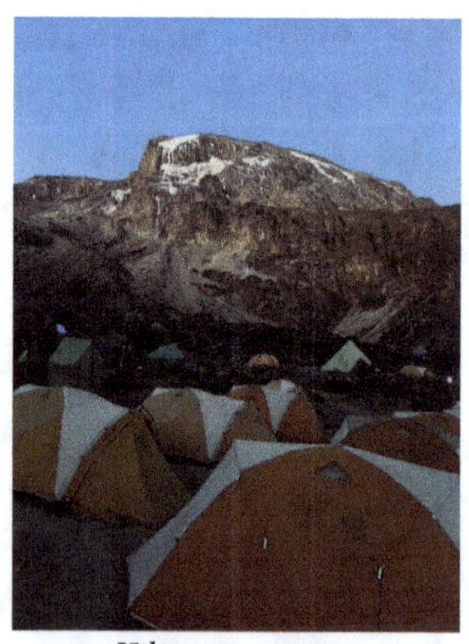

Kilimanjaro camp.

He also felt extremely fatigued and stated that every action felt more difficult. Though he could tell his body was struggling to adapt, Jonathan continued to push forward with full force. He made it to the second camp at 11,500 feet (3,500 meters).

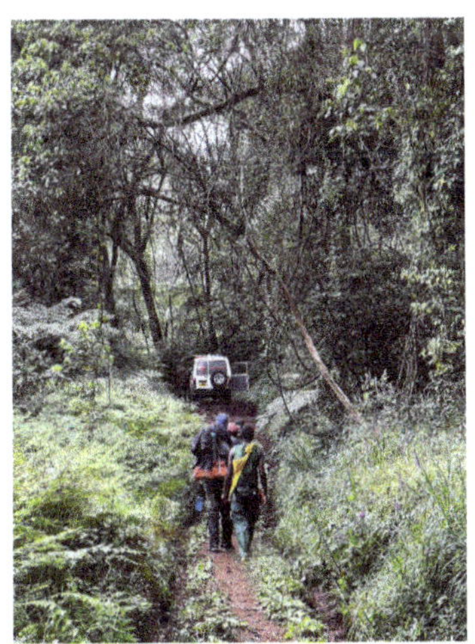

The emergency medical vehicle meeting the hypoxic climber.

"Day three, we went from 11,500 feet [3,500 meters] to 13,800 feet [4,200 meters]," Jonathan recounts. "After we arrived at this camp, our guides offered to allow us to take a break, then hike even higher. This was [an] optional acclimatization test ... but I actually skipped it. I was so tired when I got to camp on this day, I decided to just nap in the tent until dinnertime."

On day four, Jonathan's group hiked up an overpass to Lava Tower, located at 15,190 feet (4,630 meters). This was also an altitude test, and he passed. To his relief, he was beginning to feel more like his normal self, even though this was the highest he'd ever climbed. But when the group stopped for lunch at the tower, Jonathan did not have much of an appetite. He ate the food anyway at the insistence of the guides.

"Then after lunch," he said, "we descended [2,100 feet, or 650 meters] down to Barranco Camp, and this is where I realized I had HAPE."

As they were nearing the camp, Jonathan felt fluid building in his lungs. At first, it was easy to cough up, but by evening, he felt like he was drowning and was unable to lie down. The guides urged him to hike down right away but he didn't want to hike in the dark, so he spent the night alternately propped up on duffle bags and sitting in a chair. At one point, his oxygen dropped to 67%.

In the morning, Jonathan received thirty minutes of oxygen treatment before beginning his eight-hour descent. His symptoms improved when he reached 6,500 feet (2,000 meters). He was picked up in a rescue vehicle and received further treatment at a hospital in Moshi.

While Jonathan made a full recovery, he stated that he still felt the effects of HAPE at times while exercising back in Colorado, even months after the experience.

Jonathan plans to re-attempt the climb in a few years. Even though he had only been two days away from reaching the summit, he knew turning back was the best choice.

Jonathan's story serves as an important reminder to those living at altitude that HAPE can affect anyone. His wife, Katie, along with everyone else in the group, also experienced mild symptoms of altitude sickness, including headaches.

Research still needs to be conducted on the cause and prevention of this condition. While this shouldn't stop hikers from climbing mountains, they should be aware of the signs and symptoms of HAPE, understand the best ways to prevent it from occurring, and know when to seek treatment.

(Photos in this chapter credited to Jonathan Huffman.)

REFERENCES

1. Ebert-Santos C. High-Altitude Pulmonary Edema in Mountain Community Residents. High Alt Med Biol. 2017 Sep;18(3):278-284. doi: 10.1089/ham.2016.0100. Epub 2017 Aug 28. PMID: 28846035.

2. Ucrós S, Aparicio C, Castro-Rodriguez JA, Ivy D. High altitude pulmonary edema in children: A systematic review. Pediatr Pulmonol. 2023;58(4):1059-1067. doi:10.1002/ppul.26294.

Can I Ever Go Back Up to High Altitude Again? Recurrence Risk of HAPE and HARPE

If you've had HAPE, can you ever live at high altitude again? Or do you need to permanently move to a lower elevation?

To answer these questions, it's important to understand that disease processes often differ at high altitudes, and some conditions have only been known to occur at high elevations. Most of the resources I cite here refer to "high altitude" being at or above 8,200 feet (2,500 meters).

Ebert Family Clinic in Frisco, Colorado, is at 9,075 feet (2,766 meters). Many areas in the immediate vicinity are over 10,000 feet (3,000 meters), with some patients living above 11,000 feet (3,300 meters). Two of the more common conditions we see at the clinic are **high-altitude pulmonary edema (HAPE)** and **high-altitude resident pulmonary edema (HARPE)**, similar conditions that affect slightly different populations in this region of the Colorado Rocky Mountains.

With classic HAPE, a visitor may come from a low-altitude area to Frisco on a ski trip with friends. On the first or second day, the person might notice a nagging cough and wonder if they caught a virus on the plane ride to Denver. The cough is usually followed by shortness of breath that begins to make daily tasks overwhelmingly difficult. One of the biggest dangers of HAPE is its gradual onset, leading patients to believe their symptoms are caused by something else. A similar phenomenon is seen in re-entry HAPE, where a resident of a high-altitude location travels to lower altitude for a trip, and upon return experiences these same symptoms.[1]

In HARPE, a person living and working here in Frisco may be getting ill (or slowly recovering from a viral illness) and notice a worsening cough and fatigue. These cases are even more insidious because they go unrecognized, meaning treatment is sought very late. **Dr. Christine Ebert-Santos** and her team at Ebert Family Clinic hypothesize that while residents have adequately acclimated to the high-altitude environment, the additional lowering of blood oxygen due to respiratory illnesses with inflammation may be the inciting event in these cases.

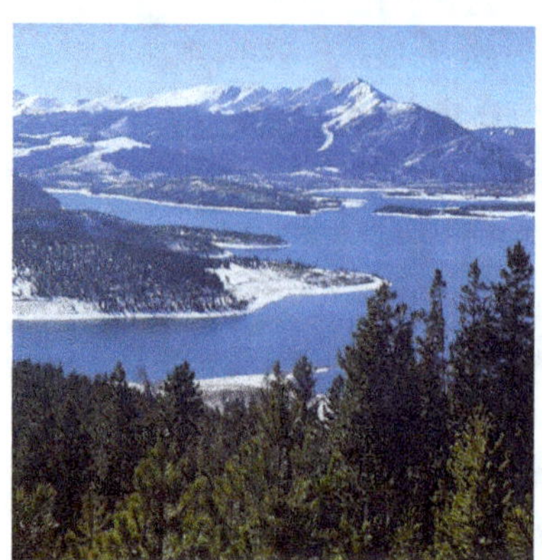

Peak One and the Tenmile Range over Lake Dillon from the Oro Grande Trail in Summit County, Colorado.

In both cases, symptoms are difficult to confidently identify as a serious illness, an upper respiratory infection, or simply difficulty adjusting to altitude. For this reason, Dr. Chris recommends that everyone staying overnight at high altitude obtain a pulse oximeter. Many people became familiar with the use of these instruments during the COVID-19 pandemic. The pulse oximeter measures what percentage of your blood is carrying oxygen. At high altitude, a healthy level of oxygenation is typically 90% or more. This is an easy way to both identify potential HAPE/HARPE, as well as reassure patients they are safely coping with the high-altitude environment.[2]

HAPE/HARPE are each a direct result of hypobaric hypoxia, a lack of oxygen availability at altitude due to decreased atmospheric pressure. At certain levels of hypoxia, we observe a breakdown in the walls between blood vessels and the structures in lungs responsible for oxygenating blood. The process is still not totally understood, but some causes of this breakdown include an inadequate increase in breathing rates, reduced blood delivered to the lungs, reduced fluid being cleared from the lungs, and excessive constriction of blood vessels throughout the body. These processes cause fluid accumulation throughout the lungs in the areas responsible for gas exchange, making it harder to oxygenate the blood.[3]

We do know that genetics play a significant role in a person's risk of developing HAPE/HARPE. Studies have proposed many different genes that may contribute, but research has not, so far, given healthcare providers a clear picture of which patients are most at risk. Those at higher risk of pulmonary hypertension (high blood pressure in the blood vessels of the lungs) are more likely to develop HAPE.[4] This includes some types of congenital heart defects.[5,6] Elevated pulmonary pressure reaches a tipping point and appears to be the first event in this process. While pulmonary hypertension is essential for HAPE/HARPE, this by itself does not cause the condition. The other ingredient is uneven constriction of blood vessels in the lungs. More blood flow shunted to fewer vessels leads to fluid leakage. As the blood-oxygen barrier is broken down in these areas, there can be hemorrhaging in the air sacs of the lungs.[3]

Healthcare providers and scientists have observed that HAPE/HARPE is rapidly reversed by supplemental oxygen or descent from altitude. Both strategies increase the availability of oxygen in the lungs, reducing the pressure on the lungs' blood vessels by vasodilation, quickly improving the integrity of the blood-oxygen barrier.

In reviewing over one hundred cases of emergency room patients in Frisco diagnosed with hypoxemia

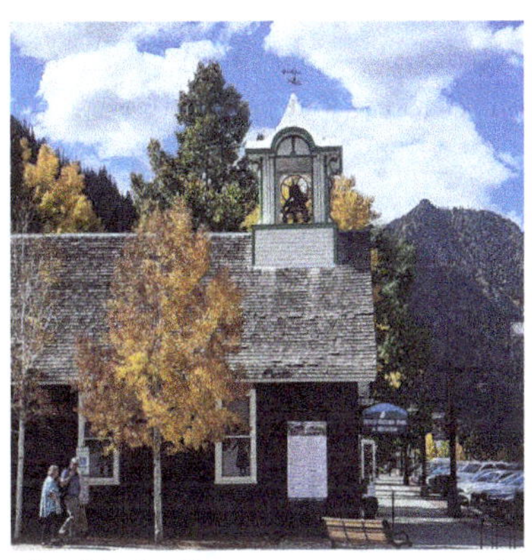

An old schoolhouse, now a museum, in the Frisco Historic Park & Museum, Frisco, Colorado.

(low blood oxygen content), Dr. Chris and her team have begun to see trends that suggest the availability of at-home oxygen markedly reduces the risk of a trip to the hospital. This demonstrates that patients with pulse oximeters and supplemental oxygen have the capability to notice possible symptoms of HAPE, assess their blood oxygen content, and apply supplemental oxygen if needed. In the case of many of our patients, this equipment prevents severe HAPE, keeps them out of the hospital, and allows them time to schedule appointments with their primary care providers to better evaluate symptoms.

Patients with histories of asthma, cancer, pneumonia, and previous HAPE/HARPE are often better educated and alert to these early signs of hypoxia and begin treatment earlier on in the course of HAPE/ HARPE, reducing the relative incidence identified at medical facilities. There are many reasons to seek emergent care, such as low oxygen with a fever. Patients with other conditions causing low oxygen, such as chronic lung disease, may not be appropriately treated with supplemental oxygen, although this is a very small portion of the population. Discussions with healthcare providers on the appropriate prevention plan for each patient will help educate and prevent emergency care visits in both residents and visitors.

A review of the case reports in smaller populations suggests that the previously estimated reoccurrence rate of 60%–80% is exaggerated. This is a significant finding as healthcare providers have relied on this reoccurrence rate to make recommendations to patients who have been diagnosed with HAPE. A review of twenty-one cases of children in Colorado diagnosed with HAPE reported that 42% experienced at least one reoccurrence.[7] This study was conducted by voluntary completion of a survey, which can lead to significant participation bias affecting the results, as patients more impacted by HAPE are more likely to complete these surveys. Another study looking at three cases of gradual reascent following an uncomplicated HAPE diagnosis showed no evidence of reoccurrence. The paper also suggested there may be some remodeling of the lung anatomy after an episode of HAPE that helps protect a patient from reoccurrence.[8] Similar suggestions of remodeling have been proposed through evidence of altitude being a protective factor in preventing death, as demonstrated by fatality reports from COVID-19.[9]

A review article from 2022 by Ucros et al. showed a reoccurrence rate of 21%, highest among mountain residents who travel to lower altitudes and develop re-entry HAPE. An ongoing analysis of 248 hypoxic children seen in the emergency department in Frisco (at 9,000 feet, or 2,700 meters) found a recurrence of around 40%, again mostly re-entry HAPE and HARPE, since residents have a much higher exposure to the hypoxic environment, adding to their risk. Recurrence for visitors with classic HAPE is difficult to determine as they are unlikely to be seen in the same medical facility, but the medical histories taken during the encounters in this study do not reflect any prior episodes.

Without larger studies and selection of participants to eliminate other variables like preexisting diseases, we are left to speculate on the true rate of reoccurrence based on the limited information we have. Strategies to reduce the risk of HAPE/HARPE include access to supplemental oxygen, pulse oximeters, and prescription medications.[10] Research should also continue to seek evidence of which individuals are most at risk for developing HAPE/HARPE.[11]

REFERENCES

1. Ucrós S, Aparicio C, Castro-Rodriguez JA, Ivy D. High altitude pulmonary edema in children: A systematic review. Pediatr Pulmonol. 2023;58(4):1059-1067. doi:10.1002/ppul.26294.

2. Deweber K, Scorza K. Return to activity at altitude after high-altitude illness. Sports Health. 2010;2(4):291-300. doi:10.1177/1941738110373065.

3. Bärtsch P. High altitude pulmonary edema. Med Sci Sports Exerc. 1999;31(1 Suppl):S23-S27. doi:10.1097/00005768-199901001-00004.

4. Eichstaedt C, Benjamin N, Grünig E. Genetics of pulmonary hypertension and high-altitude pulmonary edema. J Appl Physiol. 2020;128:1432.

5. Das BB, Wolfe RR, Chan K, Larsen GL, Reeves JT, Ivy D. High-Altitude Pulmonary Edema in Children with Underlying Cardiopulmonary Disorders and Pulmonary Hypertension Living at Altitude. Arch Pediatr Adolesc Med. 2004;158(12):1170–1176. doi:10.1001/archpedi.158.12.1170.

6. Liptzin DR, Abman SH, Giesenhagen A, Ivy DD. An Approach to Children with Pulmonary Edema at High Altitude. High Alt Med Biol. 2018;19(1):91-98. doi:10.1089/ham.2017.0096.

7. Kelly TD, Meier M, Weinman JP, Ivy D, Brinton JT, Liptzin DR. High-Altitude Pulmonary Edema in Colorado Children: A Cross-Sectional Survey and Retrospective Review. High Alt Med Biol. 2022;23(2):119-124. doi:10.1089/ham.2021.0121.

8. Litch JA, Bishop RA. Reascent following resolution of high altitude pulmonary edema (HAPE). High Alt Med Biol. 2001;2(1):53-55. doi:10.1089/152702901750067927.

9. Gerken J, Zapata D, Kuivinen D, Zapata I. Comorbidities, sociodemographic factors, and determinants of health on COVID-19 fatalities in the United States. Front Public Health. 2022;10:993662. Published 2022 Nov 3. doi:10.3389/fpubh.2022.993662.

10. Luks A, Swenson E, Bärtsch P. Acute high-altitude sickness. European Respiratory Review. 2017;26: 160096; DOI: 10.1183/16000617.0096-2016.

11. Dehnert C, Grünig E, Mereles D, von Lennep N, Bärtsch P. Identification of individuals susceptible to high-altitude pulmonary oedema at low altitude. European Respiratory Journal 2005;25(3):545-551; DOI: 10.1183/09031936.05.00070404.

PART II
ADVENTURES & EXPEDITIONS

Surviving Aconcagua: One Athlete's Close Call on South America's Tallest Mountain

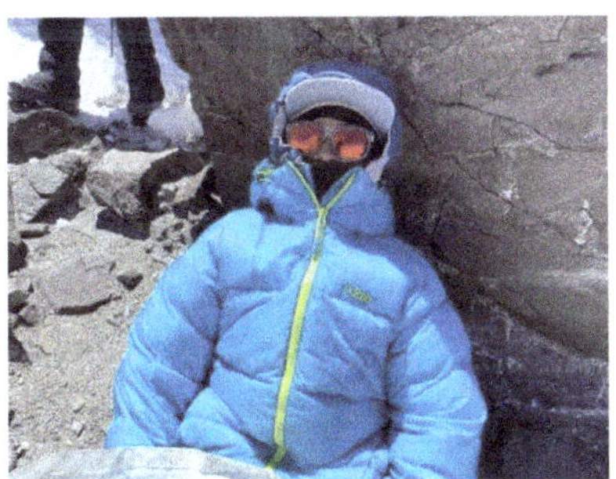

Barely able to move, about an hour above Camp 2.

"Day 10: I walked for an hour up to Camp 3 (19,258 feet, or 5,870 meters) from Camp 2 (18,200 feet, or 5,547 meters). I became the slowest person. I had tunnel vision. It was bad. It took a lot of willpower. I do a good job of not telling people how bad I really feel. After about a mile, I told them I had to stop, and me and Logan turned around. We had that conversation: 'I don't think I should go up anymore. It's not safe for me, and it's not safe for the group.'

"The others didn't go all the way to Camp 3 but continued on a bit more. Angela said she got a really bad headache and couldn't see out of her right eye. I had already pretty much decided I was devastated after two nights and two days of not acclimating. Alejo had a stethoscope and said my left lung was crackling. We thought I might develop some really serious pulmonary edema."

This is the story of **Keshari Thakali, PhD**, an assistant professor in the Department of Pediatrics at the University of Arkansas for Medical Sciences in Little Rock, Arkansas. A cardiovascular pharmacologist by training, Keshari's research laboratory studies how maternal obesity during pregnancy programs cardiovascular disease in offspring. One of Keshari's long-term career goals is merging her interest in mountaineering with studying cardiovascular adaptations at high altitude, and she has climbed to some of the most extreme elevations in the Rocky Mountains, Andes, and Himalayas. Outside of work, she enjoys mountain biking, rock climbing, hiking, or paddling somewhere in the Natural State. In December, Keshari flew down to Mendoza in Argentina for an ascent up Aconcagua.

Sacred in ancient and contemporary Incan culture, Aconcagua is the highest peak in the Americas and summits at 22,837 feet (6,960 meters). Current statistics show only 30%–40% of attempted climbs reach the top of this towering mountain that sits in the Principal Cordillera range of the Andes in the Mendoza Province of Argentina.

The day following Keshari's decision not to summit, she hiked back down to Plaza de Mulas (14,337 feet, or 4,370 meters) from Camp 2, carrying some of her colleague's gear that he didn't want to take up to the summit as he continued to ascend. Plaza de Mulas is a large base camp area with plenty

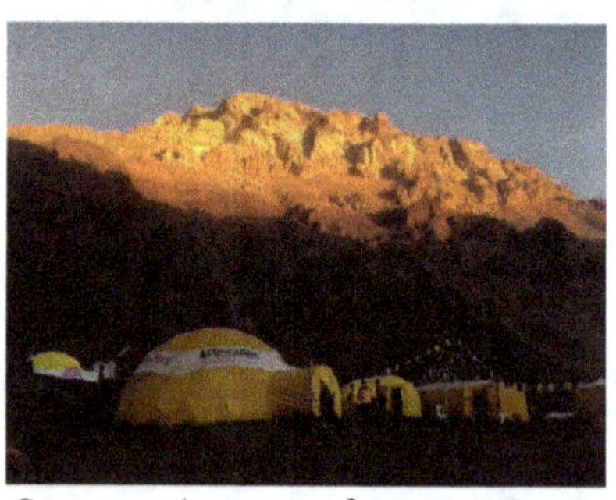

Sunset on Aconcagua from Base Camp.

of room for tents, available water, and large rocks that provide some protection from the wind as climbers take time to acclimate before continuing their ascents.

"Even though my oxygen [saturation] was low, I was functional. As you go down, everything gets better. The others continued up to Camp 3. They spent one night there, then summited the next day. It took them twelve hours.

"The day the others came back to Plaza de Mulas, everything hit me. I felt like a zombie. I did some bouldering and got so tired I had to sit down and catch my breath often, probably because I had been hypoxic and we were at over 14,000 feet [4,300 meters].

"[The next day] we did the really long hike from Plaza de Mulas all the way to the entrance of the park, about eight hours. We drove to Mendoza that night. My body was tired, but my muscles were functioning just fine. It's hard to describe."

They had done everything right and had taken every precaution.

Each of Keshari's colleagues boasted a significant background in climbing and mountaineering, their cumulative accomplishments including Mt. Elbrus (18,510 feet, or 5,642 meters), Cotopaxi (19,347 feet, or 5,897 meters), and Denali (20,335 feet, or 6,198 meters), their ages thirty to sixty-five. They weren't initially planning to hire porters, "but they ended up carrying a lot of our stuff. In the end, it just makes sense to hire these porters to increase your chance of success."

They gave themselves about two weeks to make the ascent and return. There was ample time for them to stop at each camp and spend time acclimatizing, including day hikes to the nearby peaks of Bonete and Mirador.

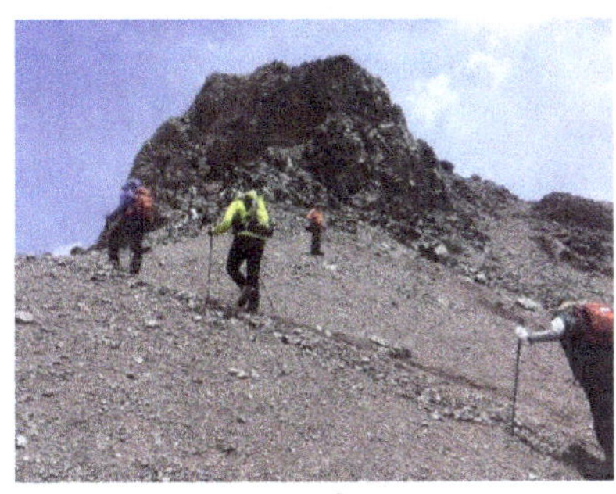

Summit of Bonete.

"Day 4 [we did an] acclimatization hike to Bonete (16,647 feet, or 5,074 meters), pretty much the same elevation of Camp 1. You look at the mountain, and it looks pretty close, but ... in mountaineering, you don't do distances, you do time. I did the hike in mountaineering boots, which were heavy and clunky, and learned how my boots actually work. You walk differently in these than a shoe with a flexible sole. The last part of the mountain is pretty rocky, and it looks like you're almost to the top, but you still have to walk an hour to the summit. It took about five hours to go up. We were walking slowly; I felt fine. From the top of that mountain, looking away from Aconcagua, you can really see Chile and the Chilean Andes."

All through their first week of climbing, and including a day of resting and eating after their hike up Bonete, Keshari was feeling fine.

"Day 8, we made the push to Camp 2 (18,200 feet, or 5,547 meters). None of these hikes made me tired. I was plenty trained. We were carrying packs, but they were still pretty light, packed with stuff for the day. We spent the night at Camp 2, took oxygen mostly at night. [My] first reading at Camp 2 was low. We were at over 18,000 feet [5,486 meters]. I thought maybe I'll just go to sleep and it'll get better.

"Day 9 was a rest day at Camp 2 because the weather was really bad. All I did was sleep that day. If you're gonna go to Camp 3, that means you're gonna do a summit push the next day, because Camp 3 is so high. You're just struggling to stay healthy. I felt really bad in the tent, but if I went outside to pee or walk around, I felt better. My pulse ox was still pretty low that day. That night, it snowed a lot."

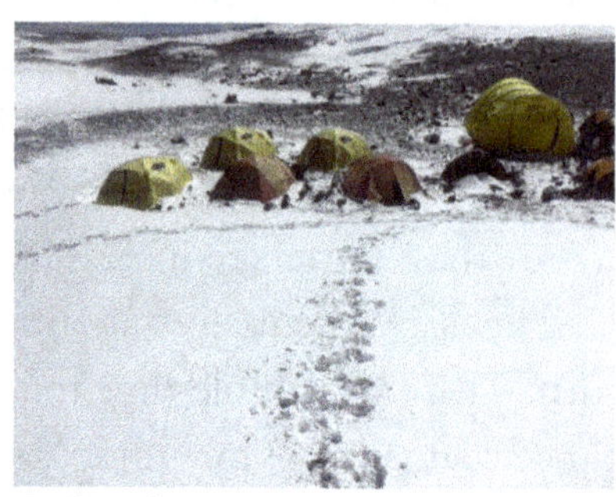

Looking down on Camp 2 covered in snow.

The day following their ascent to Camp 3, Keshari made the decision not to summit.

Since returning from her expedition, Keshari reflected on some other variables.

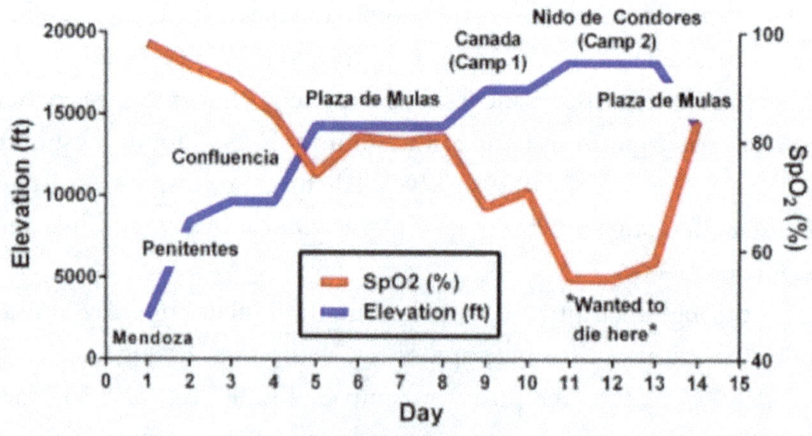

An illustrated oxy-journey.

"I swear I was hyponatremic (an abnormally low concentration of sodium in the blood). We went through four liters of water a day with no salt in the food. I was having these crazy cramps in my abs and my lats and places I don't typically get them. To me, that has to do with electrolyte imbalance. Next time, I'm taking electrolyte tablets, not just stuff to mix in my water.

"On the mountain, in general, I felt like they fed us way more fiber. In Argentina, they eat a lot of meat. At base camp, I felt like they were overfeeding us. We had pork chops one night, but on the mountain, I felt like it was mainly lentils and noodles. Even though you're burning calories, how your body absorbs them is different. They really try to limit your salt intake because they're concerned about having high blood pressure. At base camp, breakfast was always scrambled eggs with bacon and toast. Lunch and dinner were always three-course meals starting with a veggie broth soup. They fed us like kings … I brought Clif Bloks with caffeine in them for hiking snacks, Larabars."

I ask about her main takeaway from it all:

"I think I need more time to acclimate. I don't know how much more time, but maybe more time at about 16,000 feet [4,877 meters]. Maybe take Diamox [acetazolamide]. Someone suggested I should have been on an inhaled steroid, especially because my asthma is worse in the cold. If I were to go next time, I would want a couple more days at 15,000–16,000 feet [4,572–4,877 meters].

"The nerd in me wants to measure pulmonary wedge pressures via very invasive catheters. You could go through the jugular—nothing practical," she laughs. "The pulse oximeter is the easiest tool."

One last thing she'd do differently? One of her colleagues bought a hypoxic generating system from Hypoxico, "which I think puts CO_2 back into your system. Sleeping high, training low—that might have been the best thing."

Keshari went skydiving back in Mendoza the day after returning from their descent. "I was expecting a lot of adrenaline jumping out of an airplane, but there was none. I enjoyed the freefall, but when the parachute went up, I got really nauseous. Maybe I had just been stressed for so long, there was no more adrenaline left. I was like, 'Where's the risk involved in this?'"

Keshari also summited Cotopaxi earlier the same year, as described on highaltitudehealth.com.

Mt. Shavano and Tabeguache Peak: Hiking the Fourteeners

Our family has celebrated many birthdays on fourteeners—mountains that are 14,000 feet high—including an ascent up Mt. Shavano, at 14,229 feet (4,337 meters). We didn't make it to the summit of neighboring Tabeguache Peak, but I'm including it in the title of this piece because it was very much a part of our experience on this trek.

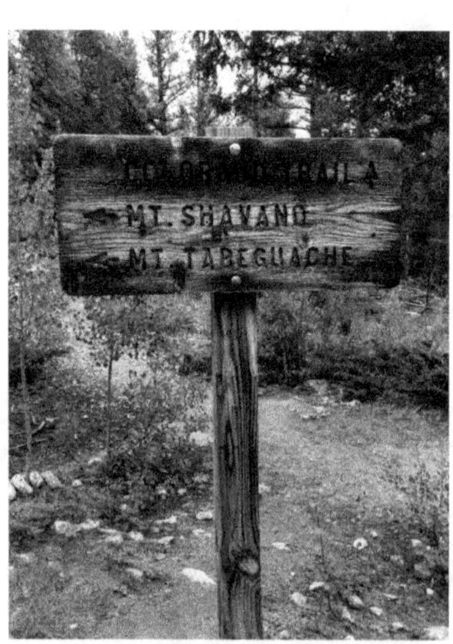

The sign, 0.1 miles from the trailhead, that we somehow missed in the dark of early morning.

The standard summer route up Shavano and Tabeguache starts at 9,700 feet (2,956 meters) outside the town of Salida, Colorado. Up to the summit of Shavano, there is a 4,400-foot (1,341-meter) elevation gain over about 4.2 miles (6.8 kilometers). If this is hard for you to picture, know that it is formidable. Additionally, the trail increases in difficulty the further you progress, and the last 0.6 miles (1 kilometer) to the top is one of the most challenging ascents I've ever done without a heavy pack.

At some point along these strenuous climbs, I always anticipate an inner dialogue about turning around before summiting. Up Shavano, this inner dialogue didn't involve me turning around so much as just passing out on a rock and staying there forever. But I did manage to summit after a 5.5-hour ascent, which included a two-mile (3.2-kilometer) detour past and then back to the very first sign indicating the trail, in the dark of the early morning, at the very beginning of the hike. As obvious as the sign should have been, I was relieved to know we weren't the only ones.

This is precisely why you should bring several resources to help guide you. In spite of all the trail descriptions with mileage that we brought, the only sure indication we had passed the turnoff from Colorado Trail was the actual GPS coordinates of the sign listed in one of our resources (14ers.com). Pro tip: you can enter GPS coordinates into your Google Maps app (assuming you have cell service), leaving off the capital letters for cardinal directions (N, S, E, W). The first number will be latitude, the second longitude (in our case, we entered "38.60218, -106.19594" to find the sign we had initially passed).

Another learning experience on this trek was regarding our campsite. We had chosen the Angel of Shavano Campground, close to the trailhead, which is outside the town of Maysville, past Salida (about two hours from Frisco). The site is at the foot of the mountains in that area, and quite small (twenty spots, first come, first served, $20 per night for two vehicles). I was expecting a lot of other hikers, all going to bed earlier than us, all waking up and starting their ascents before us, with more expensive, specialized gear, but I was surprised to find all our neighbors partying hours after we had retired into our tents.

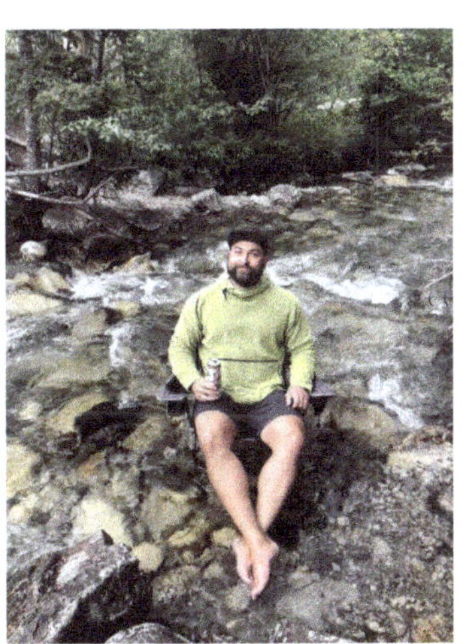

Icing these puppies in a beautiful river along the Angel of Shavano campground.

We ended up at the trailhead for the summer route the next morning at 5:15. Pitch black. Here's another pro tip: if your headlamp is dim, it needs new batteries.

Be aware this parking lot is referred to as the "Blanks Trailhead Parking Lot" on signs on the trail, and this sign is the only one that reads, "Mount Shavano Tabeguache Peak Trailhead."

The difficulties didn't stop with missing a sign that would have been perfectly obvious in the daylight. From there, the trail shot straight up. Even the switchbacks were steep enough to make me think, "Would it *be* much steeper if we just went straight up?" If you've ever climbed Peak One in the Tenmile Range above Frisco, it's like that (or any portion of that) times a hundred.

It's also significant to note this was the second time in my life I'd ever wished for hiking poles. The steep grade had me pushing off my own thighs constantly as I trudged up the incline, and my quads were burning the entire hour and a half it took me to get back down. Yes: 5.5 hours up, 1.5 hours down.

The water in my CamelBak was all I'd brought on the trail (after drinking from a couple of Nalgene bottles I'd brought in the car), and I ran out just before getting back to the trailhead. One of us had run out of water in her CamelBak on her way up to the summit. Fortunately, another one of us had packed an extra gallon of water.

As far as snacking went, we had plenty of jerky, pistachios, bananas, nut butter, and electrolytes between us. I may have even brought a chocolate-covered Twinkie. But we didn't finish all of that, and as I'd expected, my body didn't really crave food so much as liquids, at least until I reached the end of the hike, at which point I promptly finished all traces of food in the car.

All in all, I'd say it was a successful excursion, and the mistakes we made affirmed that even experienced hikers should take extra care. My main takeaway: don't rush the start of the trail. It's worth hours to be sure of where you're headed, even if it means standing in one spot, double checking all your resources and entering GPS coordinates for twenty minutes.

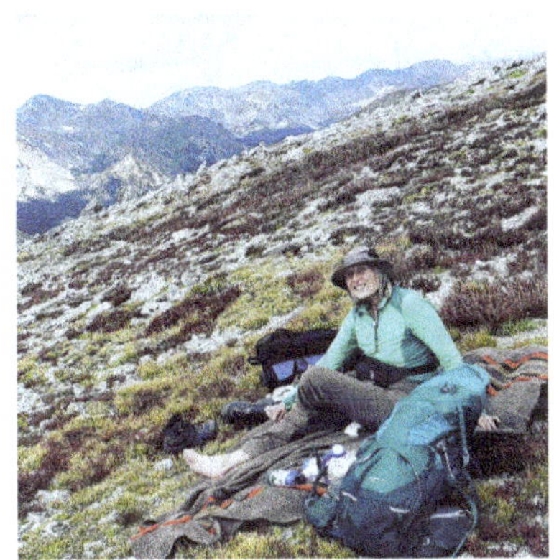

Dr. Chris, taking a break on the saddle, below the summit of Shavano.

Also notable: We started back on the right track toward the beginning of the hike just before 7 a.m., at which point it was already bright out, and I reached the summit at 11 a.m. By 11:15, all the distant clouds had amassed into huge thunderheads, and the first rumble of thunder had us packing up pretty quickly. This wasn't the first time I'd seen this. No matter how far away you think those clouds are, it takes mere minutes for them to travel. And as white and interspersed as the clouds may seem, they can collect into large, gray, stormy masses very quickly. So, beer in hand, I started a quick descent from the peak. I'd already run for my life down a fourteener in a lightning storm once, and I didn't ever plan to do that again. Furthermore, the summit area of Mt. Shavano is little more than a huge pile of rough boulders, a type of terrain called talus that requires your hands as well as your feet to navigate. The trail is neither clear nor safe, and there is no way you are running down it.

The weather was the main reason we didn't make it to Tabeguache Peak. A local we talked to on the trail, who had made the ascent numerous times, advised us to budget at least an hour each way to and from Tabeguache. It was only about a mile away, but it was a rocky, narrow ridge. And sure enough, on our way down, the hail started along with the thunder (and in my experience with fourteeners this time of year, it always did). It rained lightly

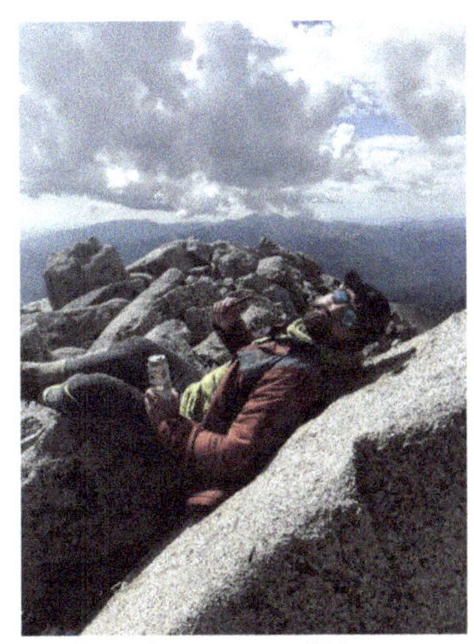

The rocky summit of Shavano.

twice through the forest, then poured torrential rain toward the bottom of the trail.

Would I recommend this trek? Definitely. It is a true test of fitness, and even more specifically, stamina. As with any other trek, and as I always strongly advise, be wise and strategic about how far and how fast you go. Elevations above 8,000 feet (2,500 meters) are when your body's reaction to the altitude becomes exponentially more dramatic, so you can bet elevations above 10,000 feet (3,000 meters) put you at much higher risk for all kinds of symptoms of altitude illness. The faster you ascend, the greater the risk. And remember, our party set out well before daylight at 5:30 a.m. In the future, should I plan to summit both of these beasts, I would certainly start no later than 4 a.m.

Paraguay Takes On Colorado's Fourteeners

Since leaving her home in Paraguay, mountaineer and hiking expert **Clarissa Acevedo** has spent over a decade ascending the highest peaks in Colorado and Hawaii. In addition to her excursions in the Koʻolau and Kahalawai mountain ranges, including Maui's Haleakalā crater, she has summited well over half the fifty-eight peaks in Colorado over 14,000 feet (4,300 meters), making her the first from her country of record to do so.

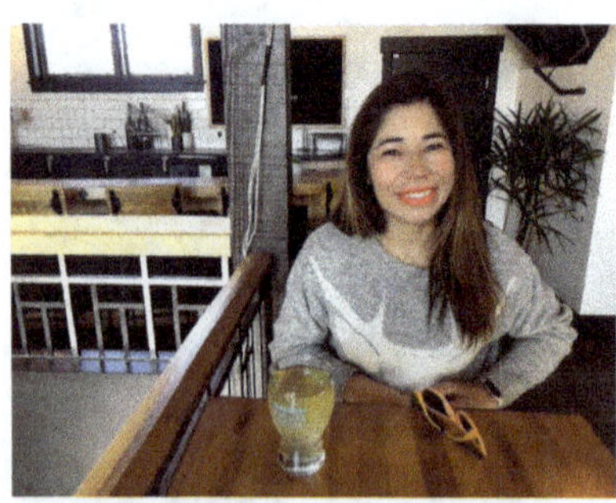

Mountaineer Clarissa at Outer Range Brewery in Frisco, Colorado.

Clarissa was invited on her first fourteener years ago when friends took her up Quandary, a peak outside of Breckenridge, Colorado, at 14,271 feet (4,350 meters).

"When I hiked that first mountain, it was hard, because I wasn't used to gaining that much elevation. I didn't really enjoy it so much because of how cold it was on the summit. Even though I made it to the top, I wasn't really having fun with not feeling my lips and not feeling my fingers because it was really, really cold. I could barely smile, and we couldn't even enjoy the summit because of how windy it was!

"[After a while] I got invited again to climb Mt. Elbert in 2012. It was actually much more enjoyable because it was with a big group of college kids from Summit, and the weather was just perfect. We were able to summit it and enjoy the day and have lunch up there. So that's what started to change my mind about hiking fourteeners, because I enjoyed my time up top. That's when I realized it's not always difficult to be up there. I think I got what all the hikers call 'peak fever.' I started going nonstop, and I met more friends that were into hiking and re-searched more about the mountain before I went.

"I always go with people who know more about it, so I started learn-ing more with other friends and other hikers. And I started feeling actu-ally great when I got higher. It was always harder to get started close to the beginning [of the trail], just to gain all that elevation. But then when I was getting close to the summit, I just got more energy. I just got more excited to be at the top. That's the goal. It's a great feeling."

Clarissa has an app that allows her to upload photos and keep a record of every fourteener she's hiked. She pulls it up and recounts year after year of summits, some she's even done more than once.

There is a system that rates every trail by level of difficulty, with Class 1 being the easiest and Class 4 being the hardest. The most diffi-cult peak Clarissa has climbed was Long's Peak—and it was also the most dangerous weather she's climbed in.

"It was a little bit late to summit it. It was not a good idea. If the rocks got wet, it could be very dangerous. There were people turning around. We decided to wait on a ridge. There were three [of us], and one turned around. He wasn't feeling good. He was getting tired. He wasn't used to hiking that many hours.

"We decided to wait for the clouds to go away. After that, we just kept going. It did not rain on us, thankfully."

Clarissa has seen her share of altitude sickness as well. One of her frequent hiking companions, despite being an experienced hiker, repeatedly gets stomachaches and headaches every time she hikes.

"I always ask if she wants to stop or if she wants something. She normally doesn't eat before she starts a hike. No breakfast. But I also carry ginger candy ... I learned that from other hikers telling me it can help settle your stomach a little bit. It's everywhere, in all the stores. Now they've created gums. I've started chewing them on my hikes just in case. You never know. I've seen people who hike all the time, and they ate something that didn't digest well, and they feel sick and get a little dizzy.

"I've never experienced any headaches on the way up. The only time I remember having a headache is when I ran out of water. I hiked Oxford and Belford in the Saguache Range on the same day. My head hurt and it lasted for that night. Now I take a filter with me so I can fill my [CamelBak] bladder. And I also take electrolytes. And I've started hiking with poles more as well, just because you put a lot of weight on your knees when you're hiking down. It's very smart to start using poles."

When it comes to preparing for such demanding ascents, Clarissa recommends staying well-hydrated and spending some time at an intermediate altitude before hitting the trail. Consuming caffeine and alcohol the night before doesn't typically help.

"It doesn't matter how fit you are ... you can still get really sick. I've heard of people who get headaches for several days because [they're] not used to [the elevation here]."

Clarissa also says it's important that you start any hiking at all to build strength in your lungs.

"It does hurt," she says about the stress on your respiratory system.

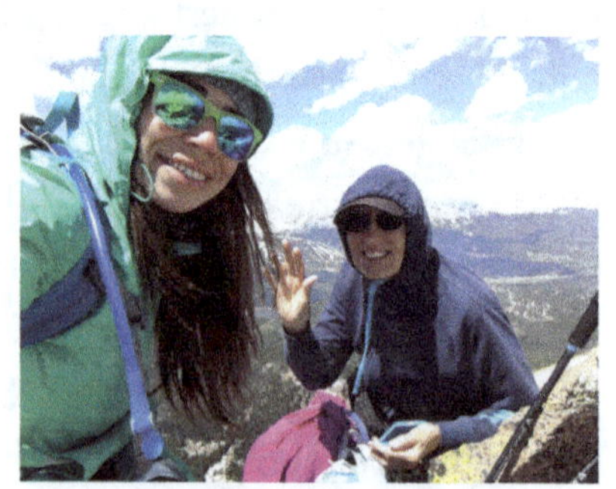

Clarissa and Dr. Chris at 14,000 feet (4,300 meters).

"I remember when I was hiking Quandary, my chest was so pressed, my heart was [beating] so fast, my stomach was feeling weird, like I had to pee or I had to do number two or something. It was such a difficult part of … gaining all that elevation.

"You've gotta find a good pace for yourself. I see many of my friends going really fast ahead of me, then they're very tired and they have a hard time getting to the top. I've waited for many people because they are struggling so much at the end. Take as many breaks as you think [you need]. Carry enough water!"

Clarissa keeps seeing hikers run out of water. "They just bring a tiny plastic bottle. That's a huge mistake. And bring food, too. You will get hungry after a mountain. It's so funny how many people are unprepared. If I'm hiking with newbies, I make sure they have everything, and they're always thankful."

When it comes to shoes, Clarissa recommends finding a pair with really good traction. She's tried some more affordable brands, but says the durability is worth paying more for. "Don't ever hike in new hiking shoes before you've broken them in. Good hiking socks also have more padding at the heels and toes and help prevent blisters." Clarissa will also double up on socks or even bring an extra pair to help mitigate possible cold.

"I reapply sunscreen on my hikes two to three times. Many times, my nose will burn. I always carry sunglasses. You're so close to the sun, you don't realize. You don't want to burn your eyes or your face. Even with the sunglasses, having a hat on top of it doesn't hurt. Even in the summer in the mountains, carry additional gloves or layers, because you don't know what the weather could be. Temperature changes quickly.

"I purchased a nice, puffy North Face [jacket] that helped me. I will always have a thin layer underneath because you get hot and cold. You're gaining elevation, you get hot, then you get cold in the middle …"

For navigation, Clarissa's main resource is 14ers.com, which allows her to download offline maps so she isn't relying completely on having cell service.

"Even though I have hiked many of them, I want to be sure I'm going in the right direction ... I just love reading everything I can beforehand. I read about the class, how much exposure, how long it's going to take. Then I download the maps, look at the maps, what kind of road it's going to be, if my car can make it up higher or if I have to hike longer."

Clarissa has heard of other Paraguayans hiking around the world. Although she has never personally run into one on a fourteener, she does meet a lot of people who ask if there are mountains in Paraguay. The highest, she tells them, is Cerro Peró at 2,762 feet (842 meters) in this landlocked country known more for its rivers and the hydroelectricity they provide for Paraguay and neighboring countries, including Brazil and Argentina.

Clarissa says she's learning more and more each year about mountaineering, and she advocates learning as much as possible about each ascent before you go. The weather may be different every single time.

"Bring the layers," she says, "whether you think you'll need them or not. And leave no trace."

After Twenty-One Years of Hiking at Altitude, I Had to Call Rescue

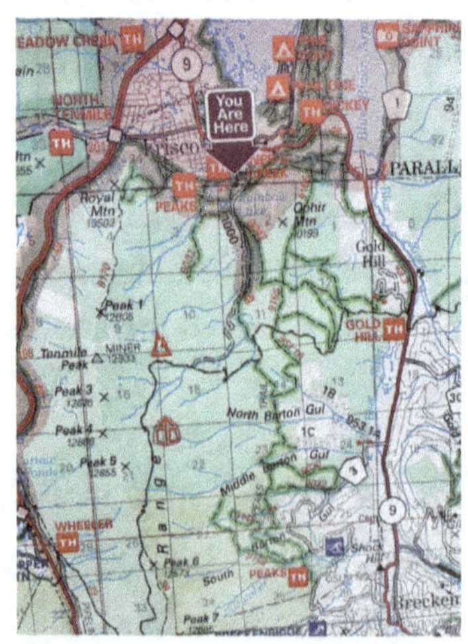

Summit County trail map.

Wild animals, storms, avalanches, cold weather, falls, fires, and injuries—not to mention high-altitude pulmonary edema and cerebral edema—are the most common dangers in the mountains. I've climbed nineteen different mountains in Colorado over 14,000 feet (4,300 meters), and some of them more than once, making for twenty-eight successful ascents. But I once had to call the Summit County search and rescue team for something I was not expecting: deep, wet snow that trapped me less than two miles from the trailhead.

It was a bright, warm day, so I had left my hand warmers at home. My plan was to hike from the Miners Creek trailhead in Frisco to the Gold Hill trailhead north of Breckenridge, which was six to seven miles (9 to 11 kilometers) one way. I had hiked from both ends in previous weeks and had seen the turnoff covered in snow with no tracks. I attached my snowshoes to my backpack with plans to turn up toward Gold Hill if there were tracks, and there were.

After four miles (6.4 kilometers), I was out above the forest with gorgeous, 360-degree views of the mountains. I no longer saw the trail markers or tracks, so I set out across the open space, my snowshoes sinking into the snow every ten to twenty feet (3 to 6 meters). The trail maps and GPS on my phone were sketchy, only showing I was very near Colorado Trail. I turned down a logging road to get out of the wind, thinking the snow would be packed. From there, I could see several open areas I thought would take me to the familiar trails that led to Gold Hill.

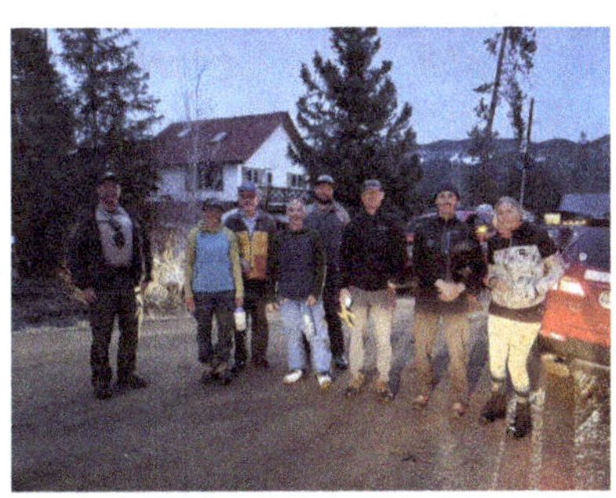

Summit County search and rescue team. Sheriff Hamit on the left, Dr. Chris far right.

After an hour of sinking into deep snow, I noticed I had only one snowshoe. I backtracked a hundred feet (30 meters), following my tracks to find it. I dug at several spots where I had sunk the deepest, but I never found it. I turned back toward Colorado Trail but could not progress, having to dig my boot out of the deep snow several times. I tried to backtrack in my footsteps but couldn't get far. In an hour and a half, I had only covered a mile (1.6 kilometers). My phone showed I was only forty-eight minutes from the Gold Hill trailhead.

I called 911, thinking they could drive a snowmobile up to get me. Bad news: the vehicle would just sink the same way I was. The 911 operator knew me, and the Summit County search and rescue mission coordinator, Mark Svenson, was in touch several times as I waited.

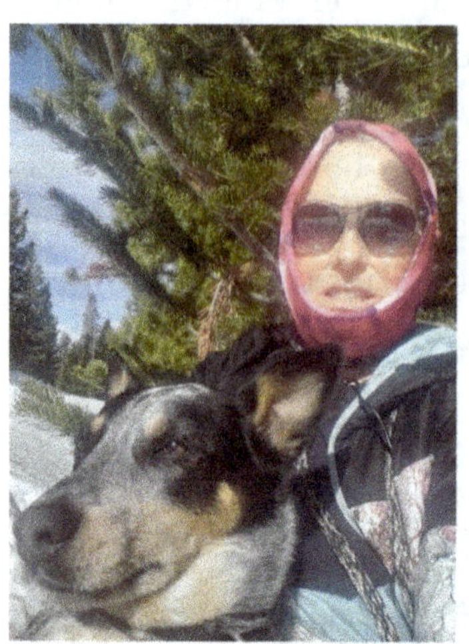

Dr. Chris with her loyal hiking companion, Isa.

I had called at 3:17 p.m., and at about 6, the crew arrived with skis and extra snowshoes. My Blue Heeler, Isa, and I sat waiting next to a small pine tree, where we found firm footing after rolling through the deep, soft snow. Luckily, I had food and water, and the sun kept us warm until about 5 p.m. My gloves and boots were soaked, so my feet were very cold, and I tried to keep Isa lying over my legs or feet. In a pocket of my backpack, I had a plastic rain shield extension that one of my students had gifted me, and I sat on that to stay dry.

The rescuers had water, snacks, dry socks, dry gloves, gaiters, and snowshoes. They packed down the trail, but there were still times we postholed on the way down. We arrived at the rescue vehicle as darkness fell. Special Operations Sheriff SJ Hamit waited with Mark and other search and rescue staff to welcome us. One of the rescuers told me how happy he was that I was still smiling when they had arrived!

What did I learn? Stay out of deep, wet snow even if it means going back the long way. Bring extra socks and gloves. Buy gaiters.

I was not afraid because I knew the rescue team was coming before dark. Instead, I felt exhilarated that I was able to do such a challenging hike without any pain or blisters, pleased that my knees were strong enough to extract my feet from the deep snow so many times, and grateful that Isa was with me to warn of any nearby animals and announce when the rescuers had arrived.

Coloradans Hike Nepal

One of our nearest and dearest, **Shelbie Ebert**, a certifiable high-country local born at Vail Valley Hospital, has been an adventure guide for the last decade. She is also a nurse and emergency medical technician. While she has done some multi-day backpacking in the past, she calls her recent trip to Nepal her "most ambitious journey to date."

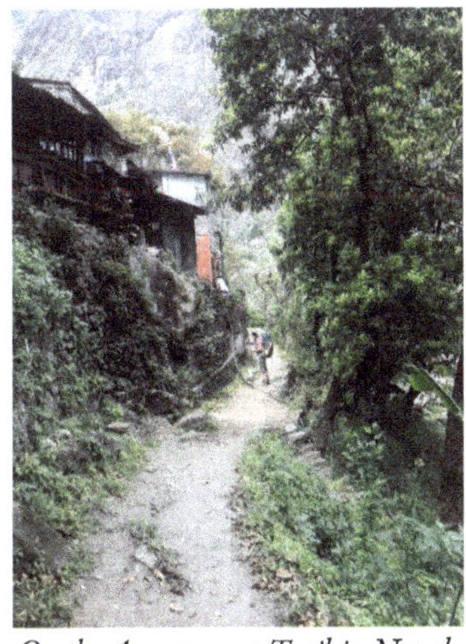

On the Annapurna Trail in Nepal.

I was able to sit down with Shelbie and her mother, Karen, and hear all about the literal ups and downs of the Annapurna Circuit in the central mountain region of Nepal, where they reached the highest point at 17,769 feet (5,416 meters).

This trek is of international fame, and there are many resources to inform those looking to embark on this historical, spiritual, mental, and physical adventure. Shelbie and Karen were in Nepal from April 17th to May 17th, but all in all, they spent fourteen days on the trail. I was especially curious what it was like for those more familiar with the unique challenges posed by Colorado's high-altitude environment.

Did you do anything differently from others you observed on the trail?

Most people had porters; we decided not to do that. Even those who didn't have porters hired a guide.

Having been born and raised at a higher elevation than most, did you notice a difference between your own process of acclimation and that of your colleagues?

I did get sick in Nepal, but it was mostly stomach sickness. No headaches or anything like that. Mom didn't feel a headache until we got pretty high up. We noticed a lot of people dropping; a lot of people bused into Manang, and from there, it's a two-day hike up to the base camp, and from there you cross the pass. They got on the trail from there. Manang is at about 10,000 feet (3,000 meters). Those people definitely struggled more.

A father and son hiked the trail side by side with us. They didn't hire porters. Shortly after we got over [the Thorung La pass], the son got really, really sick. The pass tops out at about 17,200 feet (5,242 meters). When we saw him at the top of the pass, his lips were bright blue. I think he started to get sick on the ascent. I think he was probably about my age, and he was a doctor. He had some drugs stocked up, and he felt pretty confident about doing the hike.

They started their hike at about 2,600 feet (800 meters) above sea level. In a matter of ten days, they would climb to over 17,000 feet (5,200 meters) over seventy miles (113 kilometers).

How long did you take before you started hiking?

We flew into Kathmandu, spent two days there, then took a long bus to the city, where we started hiking as soon as we got off the bus. We did take an accli-

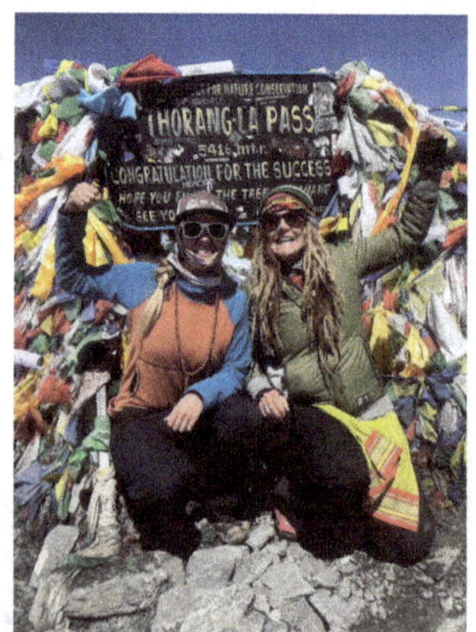

Shelbie and Karen, victorious at the height of Thorung La pass.

mation day in Manang, at 10,000 feet (3,000 meters). We hiked to it, then we spent an extra day there, about forty-eight hours.

What was the greatest challenge about this excursion?

How much constant up and down it was, with the altitude gain. The day that we went over the pass, it felt like a good day to me because it resembled hiking in Colorado. But those days of up and down prepared us well for the pass.

Did you do any training in preparation for this excursion?

No, absolutely not. I read a lot of blogs, so I knew what to expect. I tried to have just a really good plan for what we could and couldn't do, and when we got to Kathmandu, I stocked up on all kinds of drugs, because anyone can buy them. Diamox. I think I maybe only took one, once, on our ascension day, just to get ahead of the game.

Did you change or adjust your diet at all to prepare for this excursion?

I thought I did. I looked up some Nepali food online and tried cooking it at home to prepare my stomach for the type of food that we would be eating, but I found it was nothing like actual Nepali lentils and rice.

I learned some hard lessons about food. A lot of the lentils in Nepal made me sick. Luckily, they have a lot of potato-based dishes.

[There was a] surprising amount of good snacks available, [lots of pre-packaged cashews, nuts, cookies, and snacks]. I would recommend for anybody to bring five or six Clif Bars for the harder days.

Also kept some sugar on me: Snickers, chocolate, gummies ... I forced Karen to eat some sugar when she wasn't feeling well, and that seemed to improve her condition.

Karen did experience some symptoms of altitude sickness as they ascended the highest point of the trek, Thorung La.

In retrospect, is there anything you would have done differently in preparation and/or on the trail?

I would have packed a lot less. We had about 35 to 40 pounds (16 to 18 kilograms) in our bags, and that was way too much—and totally unnecessary. Less is more on the trail. We did end up hiring a porter to carry my mom's pack on our big day, and that was an excellent decision.

Did you notice anything different upon your return to a much lower elevation?

I felt really strong! I was really grateful for my body. I think it was mostly a mental shift. I felt more capable doing most activities, whether it was mental or not. I started taking better care of myself. I started running in the mornings before school, which is something I never would have felt before.

I thought, "I hiked 17,000 feet, I can probably run a mile and be okay in the morning."

Any other advice you'd give to other travelers intent on similar excursions?

You know what? Go for it! It's not as hard as you think. I came to a country I'd never been to before with a book in my hand, and we did it! I think anybody can really do it.

Shelbie is honored to have shared this experience with her wonderful, strong mother. And this isn't the first or last adventure they will have together. True backcountry buffs, I can always find them on all types of gear on the snow, on the river, or on the trail.

**PART III
HUTS**

Packing for a Spring Hut Trip

Another winter has come and gone, and spring has arrived in Colorado. Usually, this means winter will be back a few more times before all the snow melts.

We've organized a team of friends from San Francisco, Denver, and Colorado high country for a backcountry excursion to one of Colorado's 10th Mountain Division Huts. It's almost six miles (9.7 kilometers) from the trailhead, with an elevation gain of over 2,000 feet (600 meters)—a formidable trek, even for the experienced. One of the Benedict huts, tucked into the wilderness outside of Aspen, will be our dwelling for the next two nights.

Experience in wilderness trekking is one thing, but high altitude changes the game. We will be at well over 8,000 feet (2,500 meters) long before we reach the huts, so preparation for such an undertaking requires as much attention to mental, physical, and physiological factors as much as clothing, gear, and rations.

WEATHER & OTHER CONDITIONS

Everything we do will depend on the weather, so it's important to carefully track all the resources available to us. At the top of that list—in this region—is the Colorado Avalanche Information Center. They provide up-to-date reports for high-risk areas around the state using a comprehensive and easy-to-understand rating system. When considering this information, I always remember that our trek will take us through several types of terrain, and thus, several types of conditions: trees, varying steepness, exposure (to sun, wind, precipitation, and more), and all kinds of microclimates and environments, like wetlands and scree fields.

As far as incoming weather patterns are concerned, one popular and reliable forecast endorsed by people who play outside in Colorado is Open Snow. Founding meteorologist Joel Gratz updates local forecasts regularly and provides information on what to expect with outdoor adventurers in mind.

For our upcoming hut trip, it looks like the storm we're expecting will be warmer and milder than recent systems, with most of it heading toward the northern mountain region. However, it's important to keep in mind that any projected weather system can be just a few degrees colder, a few inches wetter, and a few miles closer, and conditions can change dramatically. So, let's talk about how we can anticipate this with …

GEAR & CLOTHING

THE COMMUTE

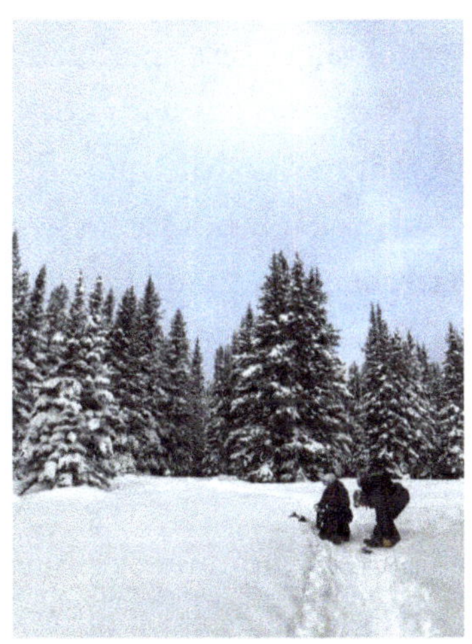

Setting out for a morning of backcountry snowboarding from the Shrine Mountain huts in Vail, Colorado.

No matter the season, there are essential comforts I always pack to get me to and from any Colorado hut that requires a hike, and to keep me happy while I'm enjoying the site. Dead of winter and height of summer alike, the sun and glare are liable to be more intense than anything you've ever experienced at sea level, while at the same time, the temperature and lack of humidity can cool your body significantly, night or day. Depending on how strenuous the commute is or how active you intend to be after arriving at your destination, you may be constantly shedding layers and adding them back, again and again, so keep it all very accessible.

For this trek, I'll be in snow gear. This is anything I'd wear snow-boarding: snow pants, outer shell on top, hat, gloves. I want it to be warm and waterproof on the outside. Underneath this shell, I want layers that I can strip down to as soon as I start moving and sweating with a 40–60-pound (18–27-kilogram) pack on. Unless the storm turns out to be much more intense (in which case, I'll keep the outer layers on), I expect my skin to be steaming, so I won't want to be in much more than warm compression tights, a T-shirt, and a light pullover. The outer shell is for blizzards and waterproofing, so whatever you're stripping down to should be significantly lighter. Also, the glare from snow is significant, so be sure to bring sunglasses or goggles. I bring both, because goggles get way too hot while I'm trekking uphill.

But here's the tricky part: what are you going to wear on your feet? This is where the weather forecast comes in. This time of year, after such a snowy winter, I'm expecting most of the trail to be covered in snow, and the storm moving in is likely to bring more. I will be scoping out the trail pre-storm, which will give me a much better idea of what to expect, but I'm preparing to have either snowshoes or a splitboard and skins strapped to my snowboard boots. Of course, skis with skins are another alternative. The chances are slim that most of the snow on the trail will be melted down, but if so, I would probably opt for waterproof boots instead, as I would expect them to get pretty muddy.

AVALANCHE GEAR

Avalanches are serious business. Whether it's on the commute or while you explore terrain around the hut during your stay, there are some essentials you can pack for the worst-case scenario. Some of my must-haves are a shovel, a probe, and a beacon, but these tools are only a small part of avalanche preparedness.

Even more important than the endless supply of technology you can invest in is knowing what conditions and natural phenomena to be aware of during your trek, and the Colorado Avalanche Information Center is a great place to familiarize yourself with these.

There is only one limiting factor to your list of comfort items, but it is considerable: How much you can carry. For six miles. Uphill. In snow.

Most of the huts in the 10th Mountain Division hut system are equipped with soft mattresses, small pillows, and blankets. The kitchens are stocked with utensils and dishes. There is toilet paper, paper towels, hand sanitizer, and dish soap, as well as ample supplies of wood for burning in the wood stoves. That means most of the weight you carry will be food and drinks.

I always pack a sleeping bag and extra pillow, because the guaranteed warmth and comfort are worth it when you've spent your day being intensely active outdoors. And keep in mind you'll want warm, dry layers—that you haven't been sweating in all day—to change into. What do you want to wear when you're lounging around the cabin reading, cooking, eating, or playing cards? For me, the answer is socks, long underwear, a pullover, and slippers, all of which I can crush into my pack. And what will you throw on when you go outside in the dark cold of night to use the outhouse? May I suggest your Colorado uniform: a hoodie.

There won't be running water, so you can't expect to shower. When you're in the wilderness for a long time and need to be discerning about how much weight you carry that isn't food and water, bathing is of low priority. But for a short trip like this, I bring wet wipes; they're lightweight and take up very little space. Same goes for a toothbrush and toothpaste.

MEDICATION & ACCLIMATION

From climbing Mt. Fuji to Colorado's fourteeners, I've noticed a lot of people bringing pressurized cans of oxygen. High-altitude research has taught me just how ineffective these are. Often, the most effective remedy for altitude sickness is five to ten minutes on oxygen, and I'm pretty sure you'd blow through a whole can of gas-station aerosol oxygen before it did you any good.

Avoid this by giving yourself time to acclimate before you get to extreme elevation. Our team will be spending at least twenty-four hours at altitude before we embark on the trek to the hut. That way, members from lower elevations will have access to an oxygen concentrator to facilitate acclimation. The specialists in high-altitude research at Ebert Family Clinic in Frisco, Colorado, always urge you to keep track of blood oxygen saturation with a pulse oximeter, a small, inexpensive, and very portable device.

Physician and high-altitude expert **Dr. Christine Ebert-Santos** recommends packing the following medications for hut trips: acetazolamide, Benadryl, ibuprofen, an EpiPen, acetaminophen, and topical antibiotic ointment. Of course, be aware of any allergies to medication in your party. It also helps to be aware of the symptoms you may experience should you have trouble acclimating. These include dizziness, nausea, hyperventilation, and fatigue.

FOOD & WATER

This is what most of the weight in your pack will be. Again, there's no running water at the hut, so expect to boil all the water you need for drinking if your own supply runs out. There are a number of compact water purification systems you can easily pack as well. For our six-mile (9.7-kilometer) trek to the cabin, I will have a CamelBak and a couple of Nalgene-sized thermoses full of water tucked into my pack.

You don't want to have to cook everything you bring, so snacks you can easily access are essential, especially for the trail. On this hike, I expect to burn calories more quickly than on an average day, so I want plenty of nutrients per gram: pistachios, energy bars, jerky. And don't underestimate the power of sugar and caffeine; the body acts quickly to convert these substances into energy precisely for this type of activity. And yes, I mean chocolate. (Fruit also contains a lot of valuable sugar, I'm told.)

While we're at the cabin, we'll have access to a propane stove, so we'll be able to cook some hearty meals. Bacon, fruit, yogurt, and bagels and cream cheese are all easy breakfast foods to pack. If you are fortunate enough to be on a hut trip with Dr. Chris herself, you will have pancakes at least once. It's also easy enough to bring fixings for the most epic sandwich you've ever had: guacamole, sprouts, turkey, ham, greens, and tomatoes. It's also an easy way to justify all the calories in the mayonnaise and mustard.

And speaking of calories and sugar, I feel like whiskey and beer were invented to accompany the warmth of a fire in a remote mountain cabin. The good news is that you are sure to be carrying less out than you did in. The bad news is that hangovers are exacerbated by high altitude, so pay more attention to your consumption than you would at a lower elevation and be sure to have plenty of drinkable water on hand.

AM I READY?

Hut trips in Colorado are mentally and physically challenging, even in the best conditions. The more time you give yourself, the better. Know before you go and don't go alone. And don't be intimidated. I've successfully guided friends from sea level who don't consider themselves athletic to destinations well above the tree line without incident.

Always be checking in with your body, your team, and your environment.

The Benedict Excursion: Testing Your Limits at Altitude

In the last chapter, I described preparing for a trip to the Benedict huts above Aspen, Colorado. After over eight hours of skinning uphill in the snow and two hours snowboarding back down, we are all home again, and I've finally cleaned all the pistachios and cookie crumbs out of my car. And yes, it took me eight hours to reach the hut.

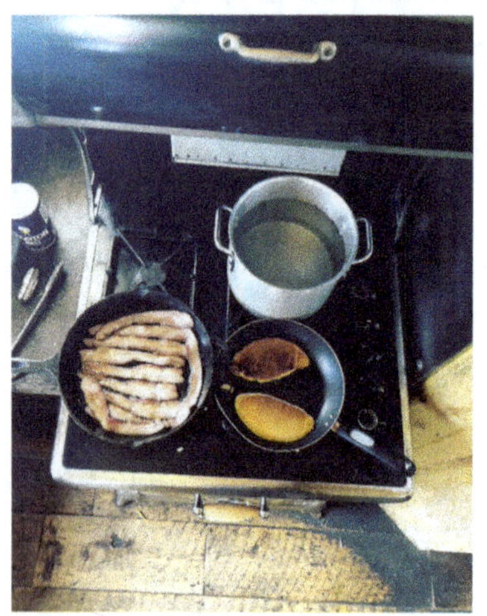

Classic hut breakfast on a propane stovetop.

I've been on numerous hut trips in the Colorado Rockies over the years, and it's safe to say the trek to the Benedict huts (there are two: Fritz and Fabi) is the most challenging, mentally, physically, and even emotionally. The winter trail descriptions on the 10th Mountain Division Hut Association website did provide some insight into navigating the route. However, we found the descriptions of elevation gains and mileage to be quite different from the route we took: a winter trail marked by blue diamonds and arrows (a fairly common trail-marking practice).

Even following the appropriate trail markers, we came to a crossroads where looking at a map, we could see the recommended Smuggler Mountain Road trail was significantly longer than the 10th Mountain trail we decided to take. And even after taking the shorter route, we hiked about two miles farther than the trail directions had described. Having started at Upper Hunter Creek trailhead, we were expecting to arrive in 4.8 miles (7.7 kilometers) when we had already hiked more than 6 (9.7 kilometers).

The trail description listed an elevation gain of 2,130 feet (649 meters), but by the time we reached the hut, we'd gained over 2,300 feet

(701 meters). This wasn't a gradual incline, either. If you set out on this trail, it's important to know that you'll be climbing at the grade of a ski hill the entire way.

Our team came from the Colorado high country and San Francisco. We were all fit, athletic, and experienced in various kinds of outdoor recreation. After collecting the San Francisco

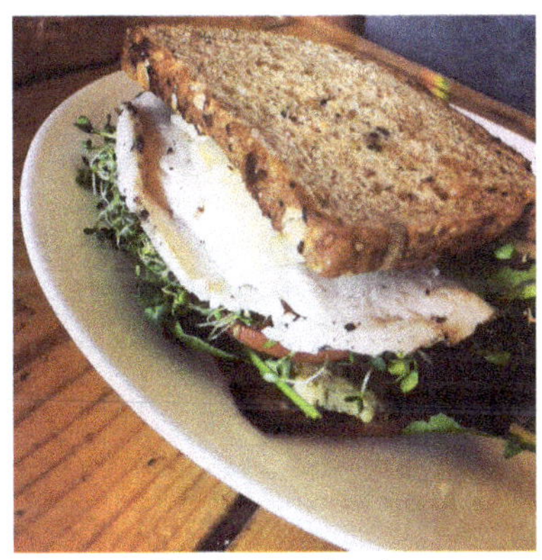

Epic hut sandwich.

contingent from the Denver airport, we made a point of allowing a full day to acclimate in Frisco, Colorado, at 9,000 feet (2,700 meters). Blood oxygen levels were quite normal for people coming from sea level, averaging around 90%. Those concerned about nausea and headaches started taking Diamox, and we all made sure to drink plenty of water and prioritize sleep before setting out on the trail the following day.

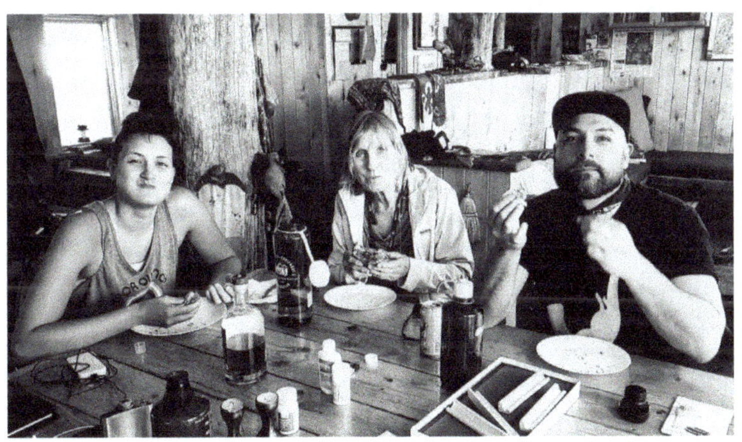

Stuffing our faces with Dr. Chris. See above for sandwich.

By the time we arrived at the hut, it was eight p.m., and the sun had just dipped below the mountains. Sore and sunburned despite multiple reapplications of sunscreen, the rest of our evening was devoted to self-care, recovery, and refueling. All the food we had painstakingly carried up was certainly worth it. Our epic journey up the mountain had been fueled by nuts, energy bars, stroopwafels, chocolate chip cookies, and a lot of water. So we immediately got to work lighting up fires to melt snow for our water filtering systems and cooking a hearty sausage-and-tomato pasta.

We were sure to feed every craving for calories, because we weren't about to pack it all back down after what we'd just been through to get it up there. Although I'd planned to do some snowboarding, the following day was mostly dedicated to resting, eating, reading, and games. Frittatas with bacon, shiitake mushrooms, Manchego, and peppers for breakfast (in addition to pancakes, of course); the epic sandwiches I described in the last chapter for lunch, and loco mocos for dinner. Plenty of chocolate, cookies, coffee, beer, and bourbon to close the calorie gap. And constant water intake. I refused nothing.

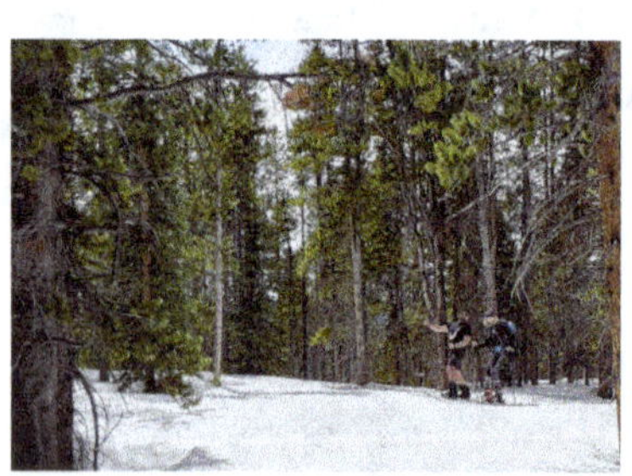

Active recovery on the slopes around the Benedict Huts above Aspen, Colorado.

Hut trips require considerable effort, not only for the traverse and recreation outdoors while you're in residence, but also for basic necessities. With no running water, snow must be collected in the winter to be melted over a fire you have to build, then boiled and poured through a filtering system. There is typically a large supply of wood on hand for these fires, but if not, gathering and chopping wood will also claim a lot of calories.

Recovery on a hut trip must be efficient for you to enjoy your time there while also preparing for the trek back out. Stretching, hydrating, feeding your cells nutrients, and sleeping are what it's all about. While most of this seems simple enough, choosing foods to replenish your supply of nutrients and treat any ailments or injuries you may have often takes more thought. As I mentioned in the previous chapter, the intense physical challenge of these trips requires energy your body can quickly convert from sugars and caffeine, which makes chocolate and coffee easy options.

But when it's time for my body to rest and recuperate, I want to feed it denser meals with better nutrient-to-calorie ratios, and this is where I look to proteins and carbohydrates, which take a longer time to process. My body will use all these nutrients, including fats, to repair and replenish itself, even as I sleep. Extreme, prolonged exposure to the

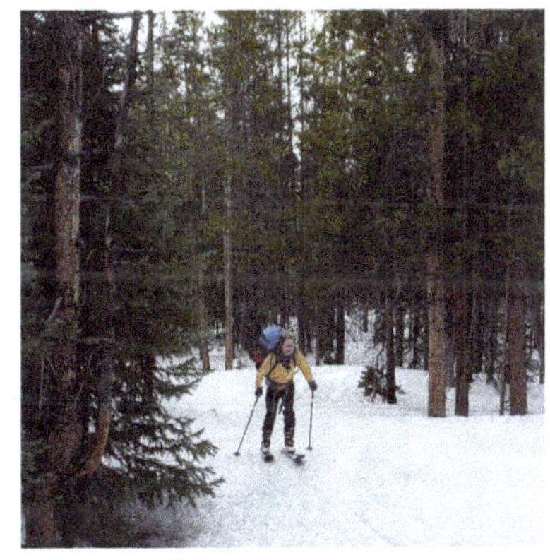

Mountain Kate.

elements stresses the brain as well as the rest of the body, and getting well-hydrated sleep is one of the best things you can do.

Alcohol, as you may know, dehydrates the body. But a hut trip without beer and whiskey is not something I've ever heard of, so in addition to these beverages, I make sure I continue to hydrate with plenty of water as well. The sugar from alcohol can contribute to your store of energy the following day, but there is definitely a threshold where the amount of consumption contributes more to a disabling hangover. I continue to do more research on the matter.

Being so sore the first night, I was a little concerned about being able to move the rest of the trip. As much as I wanted to lie down, I knew stretching was just as vital to healing muscle mass after strenuous activity, and the combination of ample hydration, nutrient intake, and stretching gave our bodies the resources they needed to optimize our napping and resting the next day.

Although I did manage to get out on my splitboard for a mini-tour around the site the next afternoon, conditions were subpar as it hadn't snowed in the area in a while, and the snowpack was very hard after so many days of warm spring weather. Our hut, Fritz, sat at the top of the mountain, so the terrain immediately around it didn't get much higher. The area was also heavily wooded in all directions, so building a kicker to snowboard off of was out of the question. The party in the Fabi hut next door invited us to go skiing, which would have involved an easy, three-mile (5-kilometer) hike along a ridgeway, but none of us felt like adding six more miles to what we'd already trekked.

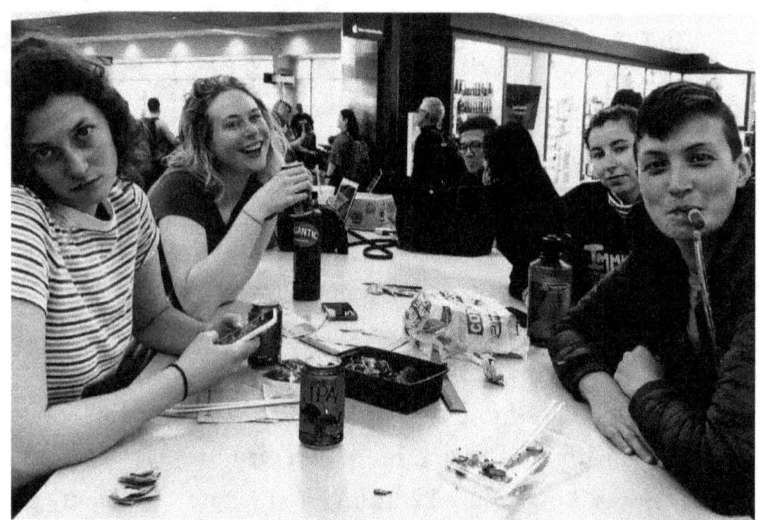

The high-altitude research team from San Francisco.

I'm glad I made a point of skiing around the hut, though. It was a great way to get my blood and breath moving around my body with fresh nutrients. One of the best parts about a hut trip is how efficiently it makes you spend your time. Even time spent lying down doing nothing is just as valuable as time exercising.

Two nights and two unforgettable days later, we set back out for the trailhead early Easter morning. We hadn't gotten any new snow, so those of us who weren't on snowshoes were skiing or snowboarding down hardpack. It felt like concrete. A two-hour ski run may *sound* amazing, but this was like two hours of squats. With a backpack on. So, that happened.

But it sure beat the hike up! In retrospect, I'd say we packed appropriately. Some extra food for the way down might have been nice, but we were fortunate the weather was sunny and warm and no sort of emergency required extra rations. Between the daytime sun and the wood stove at night, I was almost *too* warm. But again, had the weather been even a touch worse, I would have needed every single layer I'd brought. Not mad about that. In a word, "harrowing" was mentioned more than once while on the trip. But no one had to carry any beer or bourbon back.

Section House in December: Moose Country

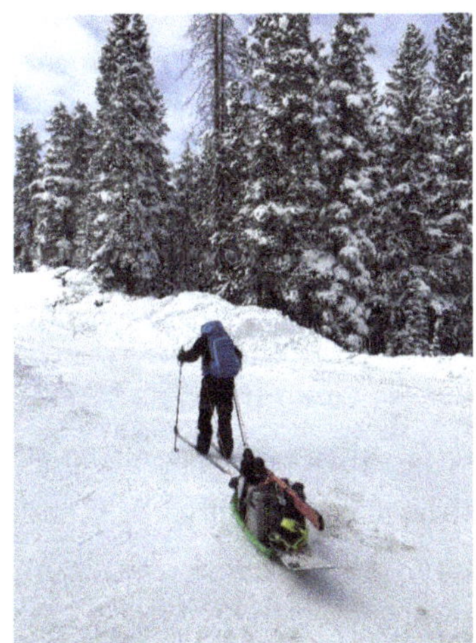

Cross-country skiing the Boreas Pass trail to historic Section House, supplies in tow.

Section House sits at 11,481 feet (3,499 meters) on Boreas Pass, just south of Breckenridge, Colorado. It isn't the highest hut in the Summit hut system, but its unique location and history are what make it one of the most challenging to reach.

Many of the huts in the Summit and 10th Mountain Division systems sit on hillsides, below tree line, which provides a significant amount of weather mitigation. By contrast, Section House is on the pass and right at the tree line, which means any wind and weather will likely be funneled right into you. And because you're in one of the highest counties in the United States, weather is highly variable.

I did this hut in a blizzard once, arriving to find the padlock on the front door frozen shut. That may have been the most I'd ever despaired in my life up until then.

Even in great weather, though, the temperature alone is a liability. When we set out from the trailhead this time, it was sunny and in the thirties Fahrenheit (just above 0° Celsius), relatively balmy for December. But the temperature in the shade can be several degrees lower, and as the sun sets below the Tenmile Range, the temperature starts to drop by tens of degrees really quickly.

THE STATS

DISTANCE

A little over six miles (9.7 kilometers). GPS and some maps may differ by tenths of a mile, so if you tell your friends six, they may resent you.

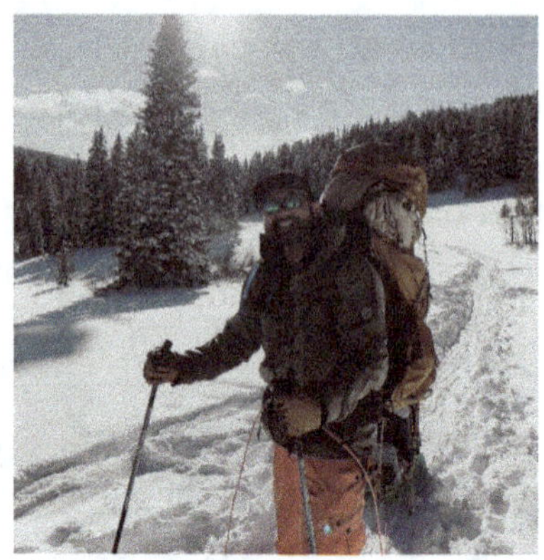

Smiling and optimistic while the sun still shines over Boreas Pass trail.

TIMING

The same hike on well-packed snow has taken me a couple of hours with no weight on my back besides water. This time, it took over an hour per mile (1.6 kilometers), including frequent breaks, thanks to all the weight I was carrying and pulling. Additionally, we constantly had to redistribute weight among sleds and backpacks to relieve shoulders and keep sleds from tipping over. If you decide to pull a sled, keep the weight low and as evenly distributed as possible. The other very limiting factor was that the last half of the trail was covered in at least a couple of feet of unpacked, fresh powder. Our lead was breaking trail in snowshoes.

While the grade going back down to the trailhead wasn't steep enough that we could keep momentum without skating, the way back was significantly easier and faster and took us half the time, even after waiting for moose to safely cross our path.

ELEVATION GAIN

About 1,100 feet (335 meters).

CAPACITY

12 people.

PACKING

I pulled a sled both times I've done this hut. I don't regret it, but even in calm weather, it's challenging at best. Unless you're going for more than a couple of nights, I'd recommend carrying everything in a backpack.

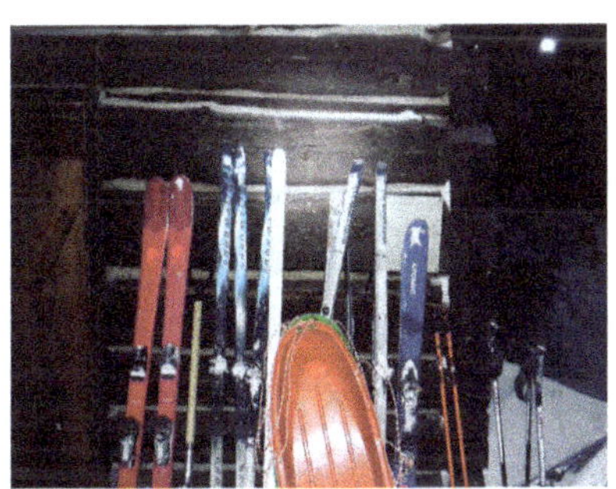

An armory of transport and trekking apparatus.

Because the elevation gain is so gradual, the challenge with weight is the distance. Pack your weight so it will still be comfortable on your shoulders after three miles (5 kilometers). The advantage of pulling a sled is having less weight on your shoulders, but after several miles, even minimal weight can dig into your muscles.

The only source of water around this hut is the snow you melt, which is why it isn't open in summer. Water purifying filters are the quickest way to refill all your containers at the hut, but you will want plenty of water before you even get there. Running out of water on the trail is dangerous. An added risk: once the sun went down on us after the first three hours, the water in our CamelBak nozzles would keep freezing if we didn't regularly sip on them.

Bring a sleeping bag. Most huts I've been to have blankets and pillows on the mattresses, but this one does not. This is also one of the oldest and coldest cabins. Built in 1882, it takes hours to heat up by wood stove, especially if no one has been in it recently.

MOOSE

Now forget all the advice I just gave you and center your whole packing strategy around how you would evade a charging moose.

This region is moose country: high, high meadows filled with willowy wetlands. Moose don't care how cold it is. In the dead of night, one of us opened the front door to use the outhouse and a young bull was standing right there. On the trail back, two different parties ran into a moose and her calf on the trail. It should be noted that moose are never in your way—you're in theirs.

But seriously, pack for your comfort and sustenance on the trail and at the hut. The only thing you can do about the moose is give them a lot of space while avoiding any confrontational, jerky movements that may suggest any predatory intent. If moose perceive a threat, they are liable to charge, male or female. If they charge, drop everything weighing you down and pray-run (pray while running) as far away as you can.

When we ran into the moose on the trail, we just waited while they wandered off our path, always staying at least fifty meters (160 feet) away. Then we proceeded with caution. But we waited for over thirty minutes and would have waited longer if we'd needed to.

SKIS VS. SKINS VS. SNOWSHOES

This was the most highly contested logistical conversation among our party. In the end, four of us were on cross-country skis without skins, one was on skis with skins, one was on a splitboard with skins, and one was on snowshoes.

The best solution really depends on weather conditions. Two weeks prior, three of us had hiked the trail in boots, on well-packed snow, after several warm, dry days. Not long before we left for the trip, however, a series of storms blew several feet of snow in, which changed everything. Boots alone were definitely not an option.

Most people who aren't hiking to the hut will stop and turn around at the halfway mark, where the historical Bakers Tank water tower stands. This means the trail up to that point will be pretty reliably packed down. But especially given the recent snow, no one could be sure what conditions would be like for the second half of the trail.

Sure enough, Bakers Tank to the hut was an unbroken trail through deep, soft snow. Our lead, on snow-

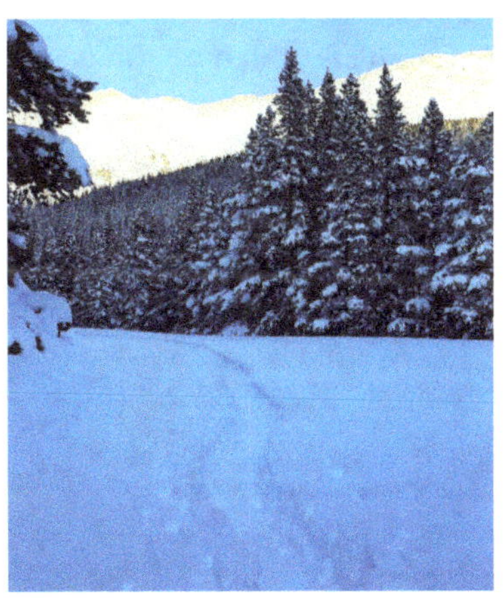

Freshly broken trail through fresh snow, past the midway point to Section House as the sun sets.

shoes, was cursing all the way to the hut as he carved the path for the rest of us. But in deep snow, snowshoes are sometimes the most comfortable option for an ascent, especially if you lack experience with skis and skins.

On a packed track, cross-country skis are relatively stable, if narrow. The boots are more like normal footwear, that is, more flexible and comfortable than ski or snowboard boots. The advantage of skinning up on downhill skis or a splitboard, however, is the width of the blades. They are wider than cross-country skis, which makes it easier to balance the extra weight.

Price is also a determining factor: renting skis or a splitboard can cost upwards of $45 a day at most rental shops, but we found cross-country skis for $10 a day at Wild Ernest Sports, above Silverthorne, and they worked well. One thing about cross-country ski boots, however, is that they aren't as well insulated as downhill ski or snowboard boots, and trekking through the deep snow required much better waterproofing and insulation than we were prepared for.

As for skins, although the trail grade is very gradual, there is enough of a grade at times that you'll be thankful for the traction skins provide. So, unless you're on cross-country blades, you'll want some skins.

ALTITUDE & ACCLIMATION

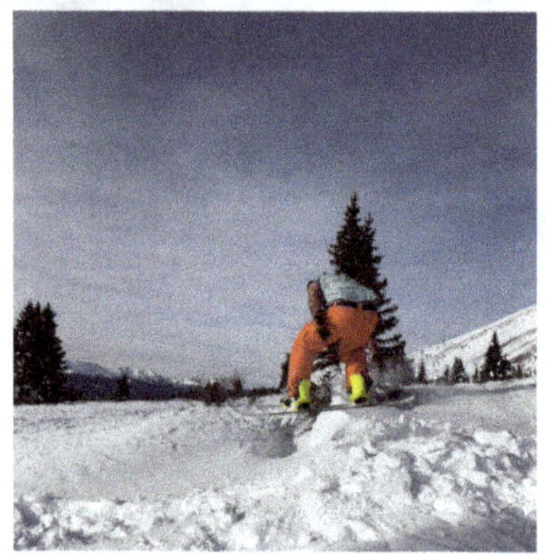

Launching off jumps behind Section House.

One advantage of carrying all the weight we did was that it forced us to make a slower ascent and take frequent breaks. These are two things you can do to minimize the effects of altitude on any ascent. In our party, all but one of us had lived at an altitude over 7,000 feet (2,100 meters) for at least a year. Most of us had lived over 9,000 feet (2,700 meters) for several years. But this was the first hut trip over 10,000 feet (3,000 meters) for three of us, one of whom had flown in from sea level two days before.

Fortunately, no one in the group experienced any severe symptoms of acute mountain illness, and I credit that to our meticulous supervision of each person's blood oxygen saturation as well as our slow ascent. The first night we were at the hut, the lowest oxygen saturation we saw was 85%, but most were between 85% and 90%, which, at over 11,000 feet (3,300 meters), is not surprising. If some slow, deep breaths hadn't brought oxygen levels up, I would have been more concerned.

As seems to be tradition on our expeditions, we arrived well after dark. But these days, sunset was at 4:30 p.m. Luckily, the weather was calm, and the trail was easy to see. Our biggest concern after dark was the tremendous drop in temperature. With no cloud cover and a recent cold front, it was well below freezing, and the only thing that kept us from actually freezing was our constant forward movement.

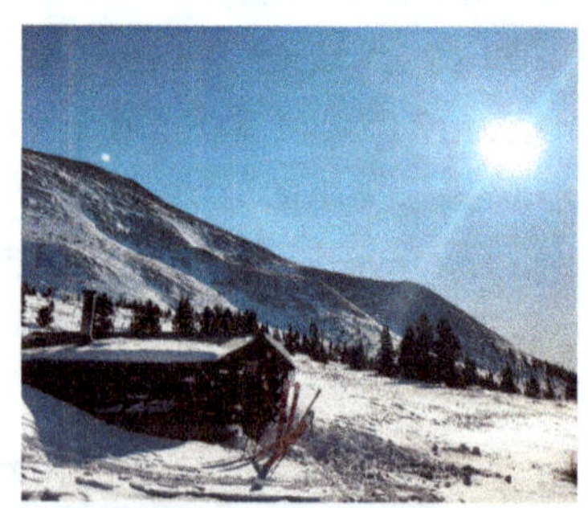

Ken's Hut, next to Section House over Breckenridge on Boreas Pass, Colorado.

By the time we had all made it to the hut and built up a fire warm enough to kick our boots off, our socks were steaming, even though our feet were very cold. It took well into the night to heat up the hut, and we all spent the first night sleeping around the wood stove. The next day was windless, sunny, clear, and warmer outside than it was inside, which allowed us to get back out on our skis and snowboards to enjoy the backcountry without weight on our backs.

It had taken us seven hours to make it to the front door of Section House, but our spring trip to the Benedict Huts outside of Aspen was still loads more difficult—and we hadn't even been pulling sleds.

**PART IV
ATHLETICS**

The Ultra Mountain Athlete

Yuki Ikeda has been a professional cyclist for the past ten years and is known as an *ultra mountain athlete*, which includes not only biking, but running races of up to one hundred miles (161 kilometers) at altitudes over 10,000 feet (3,000 meters). He has won titles in both Japan and the United States. Interestingly enough, he first came to Colorado with a plan to study at Metropolitan State University in Denver and play professional basketball.

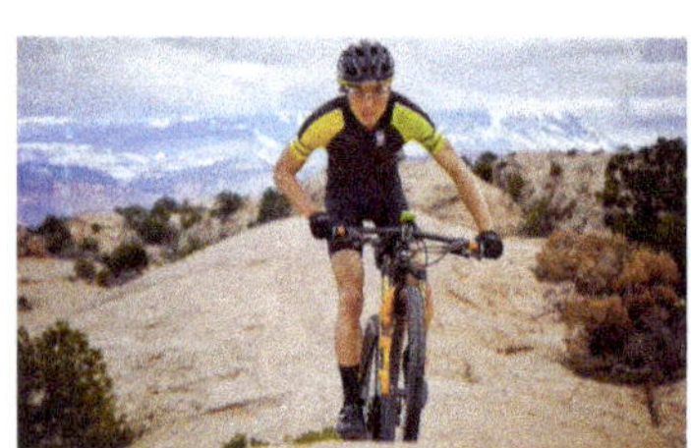

Ultra mountain athlete Yuki Ikeda.

Over decaf coffee on a warm Sunday afternoon at Gonzo's in Frisco, Colorado, Yuki tells me that growing up in Japan, he had never much explored outdoor recreation because he had been so focused on a career in basketball. Yet he had tried out for the college basketball team every semester and failed.

So he took some classes on outdoor sports, first at Metro, then at Red Rocks Community College: rock climbing, cycling, backpacking, kayaking, and others. After graduating from Metro, he ended up staying in Colorado. "At that time, I was so into mountain biking," he says. "I decided to pursue my career in mountain biking."

Yuki started racing in 2002. It took him five years to accumulate sponsors and become a full-on pro. "After every season, I sent my resume—racing results and what I do—to so many teams [to see if] they [would] accept me or not."

But Yuki started to get burned out. As he worked to improve his stats, he noticed he couldn't maintain the lead against some of the younger, up-and-coming racers. "I was mentally very tired the last couple of years. I was kind of frustrated. Last year, after the season, I was so bummed out, I didn't want to ride my bike, and I didn't feel like starting training for the next year, so I stayed away from biking. I didn't even touch my bike for a month.

"But I still wanted to do some exercise. I just followed my wife, running, then I kind of joined the local trail-running community. They showed me where to go and where to run, and I just loved it. I was so into mountain biking only, I thought doing other sports might cause injuries and affect my career. But it was the opposite."

Yuki's new love for running turned his career around. "Physically, I don't know [if it has improved my biking] yet, but mentally, it helped. Now, my training is still 60% to 70% cycling, but not all the time. When I get on the bike, my brain is still fresh. Before, I rode my bike every day, pushing hard every day. It burned me out."

Last month, Yuki ran his first ultra running race, a 50K (31.1 miles). "Last October, I got sore from just running only 5K (3.1 miles). Now I can run 50K, so that's awesome." He won.

ULTRA TRAINING AT ALTITUDE

I ask Yuki how he trains for these races. Every summer, he comes to Colorado, staying in Frisco or Breckenridge to train in preparation for a series of races at altitude. Usually, it can take him ten days to almost three weeks before he can do the same workouts he does at sea level in Tokyo.

Threshold power is key. Threshold power is the maximum power you can sustain for about sixty minutes. Yuki has a power meter on his bike that measures his exertion in watts. He also wears a similar device on his shoe when he runs.

"In Tokyo, my number is 310 watts, but here, it's almost 270 to 280. I just did a threshold test last week. So that's almost 10% to 12% lower. But still, if it's within 10% to 15%, that's very good for this altitude. But I usually take the test a week or ten days after I get here. I cannot push myself hard enough [before that]. Even [if] you've adjusted to this altitude, your power number is still lower than at sea level. I feel like I'm weak, but you have to accept it. That's just how it is."

Yuki's next race is part of the Leadman series, consisting of five mountain-biking and trail-running races in Leadville, Colorado. This next one is 42 kilometers (26.2 miles). Originally, the trail took the runners over Mosquito Pass, at over 13,000 feet (3,900 meters). But this year, there is still so much snow on the ground that the trail had to be rerouted, so the runners aren't sure what to expect. The race starts at over 10,000 feet (3,000 meters).

To train for this, Yuki has been running and biking six days a week. Every morning, he measures his blood oxygen saturation using a pulse oximeter. The first morning he arrived in Frisco, it was at 92%. After a couple of weeks of acclimation and training, it's pretty reliably at 96% every morning.

PACING

Yuki feels the most difficult part about running these long races is pacing. His coach encouraged him to run "negative splits," which involves increasing speed toward the end of the race. "At my first 50K race, even though I won it, I could have paced myself better. I just went too hard at the beginning [to] take the lead and paid for it later in the race. I was so trashed after the race, I couldn't even stand and walk.

"My coach is saying to be careful about [hitting the wall] at altitude. It's so hard to recover. It takes almost five times longer than at sea level. I need to pace myself, especially for running a hundred miles [161 kilometers]," Yuki says, referencing the race he's preparing for: the Leadville Trail 100 Run, a course of one hundred miles at altitude. "I'm so excited, but at the same time, I'm so nervous. Even finishing is questionable at this point."

ACCLIMATION

Yuki's secret to acclimating comfortably and quickly is movement. In order to get more oxygen to his body, he has to get his circulation going, which is why he feels the effects of elevation more when he's sedentary. "The first week, I feel better when I exercise than when I just sit [around]."

Also, beets. And red bell peppers. And arugula.

Yuki eats a limited portion of these

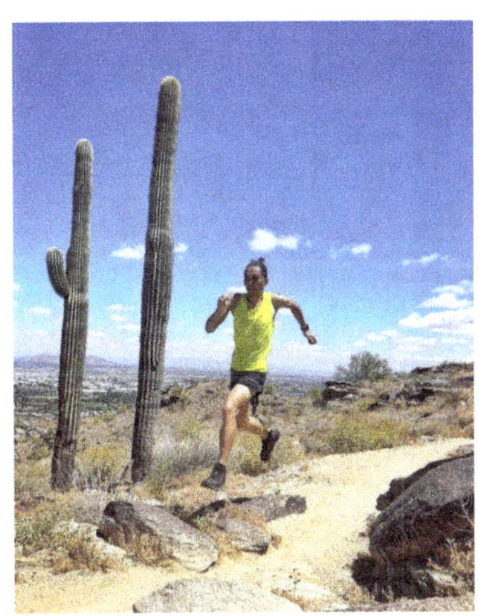

Yuki, training through the high desert.

every day he's at altitude. These vegetables provide a lot of nitrates, which the body processes into nitric oxide, facilitating blood circulation. At altitudes over 8,000 feet (2,500 meters), where you have access to about two-thirds of the oxygen available in the air at sea level, the key to supplementing the oxygen your body requires is increased blood flow. After a certain amount of time, your body starts creating more oxygen-carrying red blood cells to counter the deficit, so getting the blood moving is literally vital.

According to high-altitude growth and development expert **Dr. Christine Ebert-Santos**, nitric oxide is often the way newborn babies with complications are treated. Hypoxia (the state of receiving less oxygen than is normal at sea level) causes pulmonary vessels (in the lungs) to constrict. Putting these infants on nitric oxide gas dilates the pulmonary arteries and improves some types of respiratory distress.

There are powder versions of these essential nutrients, including BeetElite, Yuki's product of choice, which he'll add to his sports drinks in addition to consuming about an ounce (28 grams) of roasted beets. But portion control is also important, as too much nitrate can have a negative effect on the body.

RUNNING RECOVERY

Yuki has to deal with an interesting phenomenon when it comes to his ultra running races: it's tough on his guts. "I think my guts are more tired," he says, "because your body is bouncing so much from running." Yet he doesn't typically change anything about his diet for recovery after a long event.

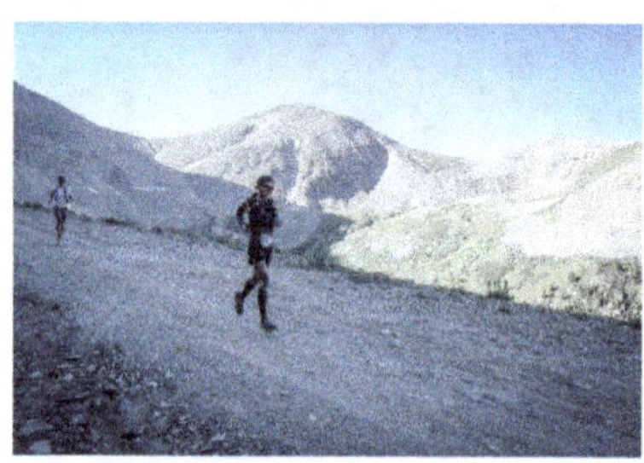

On the Leadville Series trail, above 10,000 feet (3,000 meters).

While running these incredible distances, Yuki fuels his body with an energy gel every twenty to thirty minutes. "It usually has about 100 to 120 calories. It's a dense energy. Then you take them for five hours, continuously, so it also tires out your guts. During the race, you have to maintain your blood sugar and keep your muscles moving. My muscles are tired, but also, my intestines and stomach are tired.

"Even water is hard on my stomach [after running a race]. I'm kind of worried about running fifty and one hundred miles [80 and 161 kilometers]. I'm not only worried about my legs, but even my stomach. I'm not used to [consuming] energy for twenty hours, eating and running at the same time."

SLEEP

In Japan, hot springs and bathing are a huge, sacred part of the recovery and health ritual. Yuki takes a hot bath almost every day, "especially in winter," he says. "It helps me to sleep at night."

Yuki finds it hardest to fall asleep during the first week at altitude in Colorado. "I used to take one or two melatonin capsules every night, but it's hard to tell if it helped. I just go to bed early, like eight or nine, even if I cannot fall asleep. I just take the time to lay down and recover. [I try to sleep] at least seven to eight hours a night, but sometimes it's hard. If I can't get that amount of sleep, I usually take a nap after training."

This may sound obvious, but sleep is the body's way of recovering, both mentally and physically, and sleep experts and studies have proven that the body and brain visibly deteriorate after enough sleep deprivation. And at altitude, with less oxygen available to supply a body in constant motion, sleep is more important than ever.

PLANT-BASED NUTRITION

"When I used to like and eat animal products a lot, my recovery time was slower than now," Yuki says. "It was hard to digest animal fats. I believed that they had a lot of good protein, but it was so hard on your body and digestive system. It took time to change my diet, but I now feel more

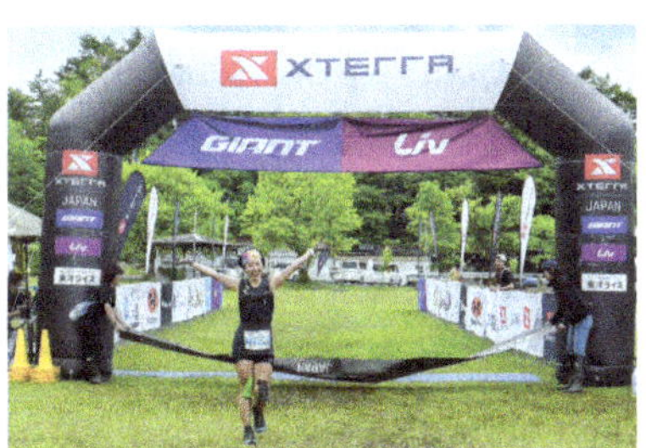

Altitude athlete and nutritionist Sayako Ikeda.

comfortable with my plant-based diet, physically and mentally."

Yuki isn't the first high-altitude athlete I've spoken to who advocates for a plant-based lifestyle. Recently, skier and duathlete **Cierra Sullivan** told us about how a plant-based diet seems to make a big difference for her, too.

LIVE HIGH, TRAIN LOW

"Live high, train low" is a common refrain among high-altitude athletes.

"One of my sponsors has an altitude tent," Yuki says. "They leased it to me before the competition, so I used it for about a month. I slept in the tent, set at about 3,000 meters [10,000 feet], then I trained at sea level. I think it helped a bit, but it might be too short to tell. It tired me [out], though. I think I needed to do it longer before the competition, like, two or three months. I couldn't train well because I felt tired all the time. But I think for altitude training, I think this elevation is almost too high. Because you cannot push to your maximum potential. For example, for cycling, I can push up to 1,000 to 1,200 watts at sea level, but I cannot hit that number here, so I cannot train in that range here. I can lose that high power if I stay longer here. But it depends on your [goal]. My [goal] is winning the Leadman series. That's why I've come here to train."

When training at altitude, Yuki will lift weights once a week "to maintain my high power." With such limited access to oxygen, athletes up here can't reach the same "punching power" that they can at lower elevations, so lifting may help maintain that power. "Very short, maybe forty-five minutes once a week, just to maintain. Weightlifting is still supplemental for your specific sport, so I don't want it to affect my training on my bike or running. For race week, I don't lift weights, because lifting weights takes time to recover."

KEEPING IT FUN

"My trick to keep going, the best way to improve yourself," Yuki adds, in a final reflection, "is to keep it fun. If you're not having fun, I think that's not good. Last year, I almost lost my motivation as an athlete. I almost thought about quitting racing, but I still love the sport. Trail running helped me mentally and physically, and my motivation came back, even for cycling. Having fun is the key to keeping going."

SUMMER 2025

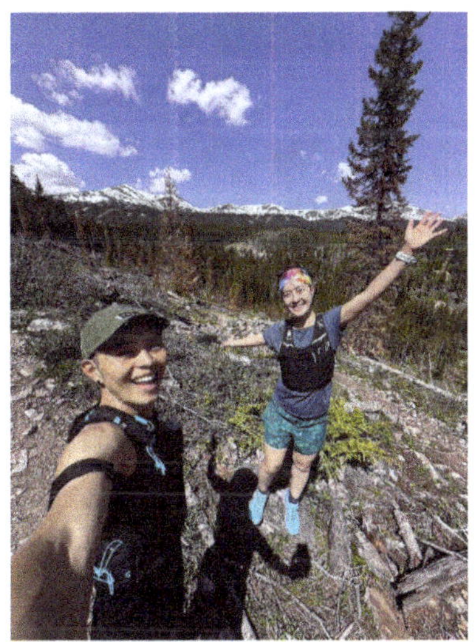

Sayako and Yuki, training together in the Colorado Rockies.

This summer, I had the pleasure of catching up with this extraordinary athlete and his wife, Sayako, a dietitian and high-altitude runner herself, who inspired Yuki to compete as a runner as well as a cyclist. The pair had been spending summers in the Colorado high country every year to train and compete before returning to their home in Japan, where they continued to compete year-round. Between their training and racing experience and nutritional expertise, they make a formidable team.

Six years ago, we were all three of us in our thirties, and when I asked about what has changed about training and acclimating to the altitude since then, there was certainly a consensus about how it hasn't gotten easier now that we are all in our forties. A significant part of their strategy for success has always been nutrition, and at this elevation, maximizing the delivery of oxygen throughout the body makes a huge difference. In our last interview, Yuki talked about incorporating foods rich in nitrates, like red bell peppers, arugula, and beets. These facilitate the body's production of nitric oxide, and they are still a big part of their diet.

Something else they've been paying closer attention to lately is iron, also a critical component of blood. It's dangerous for iron levels to be too high, but it can be a critical supplement for healthy circulation. In the case of long-distance runners, blood vessels can take a considerable beating as feet hit ground over and over again for long periods of time. One food in particular that contains a high level of iron is clams. In Japan and the Pacific, *asari*, also known as the Manila clam or Japanese cockle, is a regular part of the cuisine and easy to find. Here in the middle of the Rockies, however, Yuki and Sayako have resorted to buying canned clams to supplement their iron.

Every summer, the couple comes to the Rockies to train and compete. Their full-time residence is at sea level in Tokyo, Japan, which means each trip to Colorado involves a dramatic and quick ascent to high elevation. The decrease in available oxygen prompts the body to create more red blood cells to carry oxygen throughout the body, a process that requires more iron.

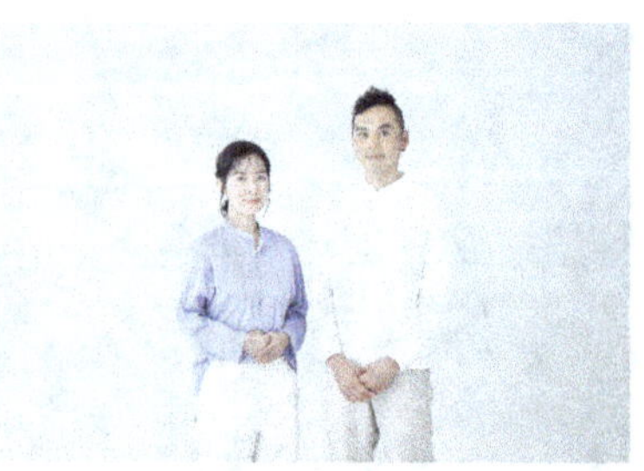

High-altitude athletes Sayako and Yuki Ikeda.

Additionally, the two athletes are paying special attention to nutrient absorption. Most of their diet is plant based, and until recently, Yuki has been eating a completely vegan diet. Organic compounds found in plants called tannins and polyphenols, while beneficial, can inhibit the body's absorption of nutrients by up to 90%. So consuming something with these compounds along with your meal may dramatically decrease the benefits of nutrition in the food you're eating. Coffee contains these compounds, so Sayako recommends waiting at least an hour after a meal to have a cup of coffee in order to maximize nutrient uptake. By contrast, vitamin C enables *greater* absorption, so consuming it (even in other foods such as citrus) with a meal can be very helpful.

"Iron is also necessary for the hypoxia-inducible-factor (HIF) pathway, cellular energy production, myoglobin function (the muscle oxygen acceptor), and thyroid hormone function," write DeLoughery and DeLoughery in a recent article for the Wilderness Medical Society. "The HIF pathway is the key regulator of the body's response to hypoxia. Typically, the HIF-1 and HIF-2 proteins are rapidly degraded, but they are stabilized by hypoxic conditions when prolyl hydroxylase, which tags the HIF proteins for degradation, is inhibited. When stabilized, the HIF proteins function as transcription factors that coordinate the synthesis of various proteins essential for the body's response to hypoxia. Prolyl hydroxylase requires iron to function, and with a low iron level, this is less effective, leading to an exaggerated response to hypoxia."

It is also important to note that, as Yuki and Sayako point out, it can take three to four weeks for anyone to experience noticeable results from any change in diet and nutrition. Keeping this in mind, it is advisable to increase iron intake weeks ahead of a trip to a high-altitude environment, although further research may be needed to recommend just how much.

REFERENCES

1. DeLoughery, MD, Emma P. Emma P. DeLoughery, MD and Thomas G. DeLoughery, MD, "Women, Iron, and Altitude—Path to the Peak," Wilderness Medical Society 2025.

Pre-acclimatization: A Synopsis of Dr. Peter Hackett's Lecture at the Wilderness Medical Society

What is **pre-acclimatization**? It is a process of adjusting to a new climate, usually a higher elevation, reducing hypoxemia in high-altitude settings to ease altitude sickness and save time and money. It can also allow for better sleep, enhanced comfort, and improved physiological and cognitive performance at high altitudes. Acclimatization is a time-dependent process, as over 5,000 genes are impacted by a large shift in elevation, affecting ventilation, plasma volume, and hemoglobin mass, among other things.

The whole process is not completely understood, but one key element is the *hypoxic ventilatory response* (*HVR*), which is when the aortic artery baroreceptors trigger an increase in respiration as oxygen in the blood decreases. This happens immediately as you ascend in altitude and maximizes seven to fourteen days later. Arterial oxygen increases with increased ventilation/saturation and dropping plasma volume, increasing hemoglobin concentration, then later on increasing overall hemoglobin production, which in theory reduces altitude sickness.

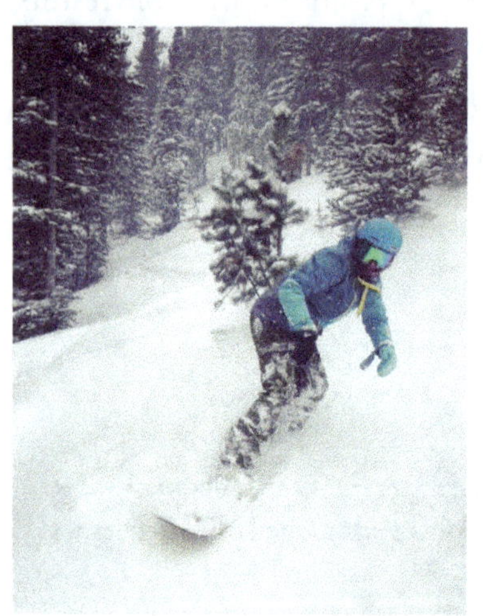

A powder day in Breckenridge, Colorado, above 10,000 feet (3,000 meters).

So how can you prepare yourself for travel to higher altitudes?

Some of the better-known methods of pre-acclimatization are spending time at higher altitudes prior to reaching your destination, using a hyperbaric or normobaric chamber, blood doping, hypoxic exercise training, and assorted pharmaceutical methods. All of these are options, but the key question is, which ones truly work?

Pre-acclimatization with actual altitude is the most useful. Start by choosing the maximum sleeping altitude at your destination and decide on an ascent profile that will allow you to slowly work your way up to that altitude. This exercise is most useful when spread out over at least a week, and should be completed no more than one or two weeks prior to travel so that any acclimation gains don't wane prior to your trip.

Simulated altitude is another option. This might involve hypoxic tents, hypoxic rooms or homes, hypoxic exercise chambers, and hypoxic masks. Out of these four, hypoxic tents, rooms, or homes, where exposure is over a long duration, are by far the most effective. Hypoxic masks and exercise chambers are not as effective, as their short duration does not give the body enough time to adjust properly. Although they might be beneficial in respiratory muscle training and performance, they do little in the way of pre-acclimatizing your body.

Studies show more benefit from hypobaric over normobaric hypoxia training, but keep in mind studies are very limited and warrant much further research. Minimum requirements for simulating altitude include one week of exposure for seven hours a day, a minimum effective altitude of 2,200–2,500 meters (7,200–8,200 feet), and being no more than 1,500–2,000 meters (4,900–6,500 feet) below your target sleeping altitude. Shorter-term protocols can attenuate altitude sickness, but not at the incidence some studies suggest. As to why hypobaric methods are more effective than normobaric methods, no one really knows yet, and more research is needed.

Exposure to altitude over many years by living permanently at a higher elevation, or *moderate altitude residence* (*MAR*), is the most effective method of acclimatizing, according to some studies, but this is far from feasible for most. There are studies that show epigenetic changes for those who relocate to higher elevations for long periods. These appear to be much less pronounced than for those who have genetically adapted to higher elevations over generations, but still more effective than the previously mentioned short-term options.

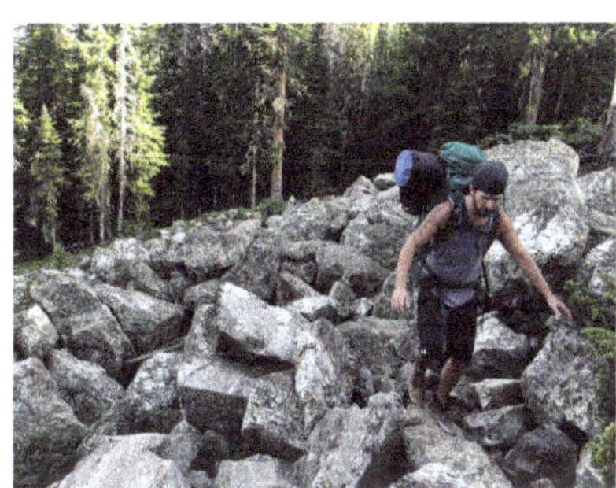

Carefully navigating a skree field on the South Willow Falls trail above Silverthorne, Colorado.

Oxygen saturation is maximal at eleven days of exposure to a specific elevation. Diamox (acetazolamide) increases ventilation and can help with acclimatization, but there isn't much data on how using this pharmaceutical compares to other methods mentioned. World-renowned high-altitude expert and pioneer **Dr. Peter Hackett** theorizes its effectiveness may fall just short of MAR, but again, more research is needed. Short-term altitude exposure shows benefits at seven days, but a longer exposure, such as fifteen days, has been shown to be much more beneficial.

Blood doping with EPO (erythropoietin) can be somewhat effective with treatment over four weeks or more. It can potentially decrease acute mountain sickness and increase exercise performance, but the data is limited and conflicting on this. It is only effective up to 4,300 meters (14,100 feet), as arterial oxygen content is not the determining factor for sleep and cognition performance at high altitudes, but rather oxygen delivery, which is affected by hematocrit and viscosity of blood.

Hypoxia inducible factor (*HIF*) is a regulatory factor in cells that responds to a reduction in oxygen, causing changes in about 5,000 different genes to help the body adjust to meet oxygen requirements. We may be able to pharmaceutically activate this factor prior to arrival at destination, allowing patients to acclimatize to higher elevations with fewer complications and better results. Currently, there are some drugs in trials, but nothing specifically FDA approved.

Data and studies are limited, but currently, the most effective pre-acclimatization method is long-term altitude training (real or simulated). If possible, plan your ascent trip to be slow and steady to obtain best results with the least complications.

Watch Out for Flying Discs: How High Altitude Changes Flight

Have you ever played disc golf? Maybe you know someone who has. Or maybe you've seen it from a distance. Perhaps you've walked through a park or along a hiking trail and noticed a warning sign: "You Are Now Entering a Disc Golf Course—Watch Out for Flying Discs." It can be a dangerous sport.

It's just like golf, but with frisbees. Instead of putting your ball into a hole in the ground, you throw your disc into an odd-looking metal basket situated on top of a pole with a bunch of chains hanging from it. Maybe you've seen one such basket on your stroll through the park and thought, "What is that thing?" That's disc golf.

I learned to play this game in the forests and hills of Northern California, close to sea level. But Colorado is home to some of the best disc golf courses in the country, so I was excited to venture out and experience them after moving here. However, I could tell immediately that something was wrong the first time I played a round in Summit County—my discs were not flying like they used to!

It was throwing my game off. I had quickly learned that life at over 9,000 feet (2,700 meters) had all sorts of challenges not faced by sea-level dwellers. After a few rounds of disc golf up here—and feeling like I had to learn how to play all over again—I wondered if my new high-altitude environment had something to do with why my discs were misbehaving.

I set out to better understand the physics behind how discs fly through the air and how altitude affects these characteristics.

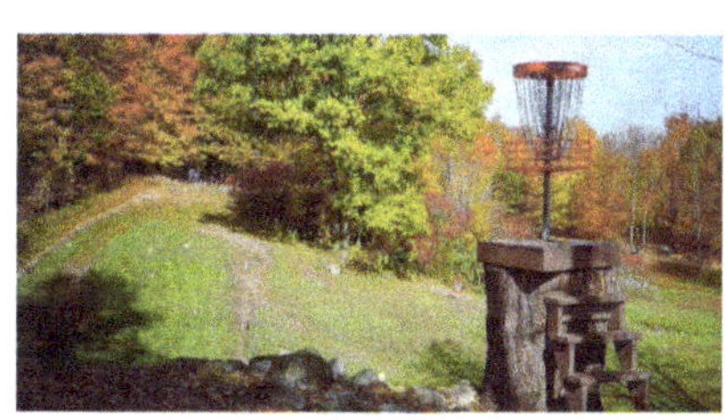
Disc golf goal.

A lightweight disc traveling through the air is very sensitive to the atmosphere. At sea level, air density is higher, so flying objects encounter more air resistance. As elevation increases, air density decreases, and flying objects encounter less resistance. So yes, high altitude does cause flying objects to fly differently, but there's a lot more to the story when it comes to disc golf.

Disc golf is a challenging game. The goal is to throw a one-third–pound (0.2-kilogram) plastic disc hundreds of feet through the air, over rough terrain, in such a way that it avoids trees, hills, and ponds, and lands in that odd metal basket. And hopefully doing so in fewer throws than your friends.

The fun part is throwing the disc *far*. Flying discs can travel much, much farther than most other objects thrown by hand, such as baseballs and footballs. The world record for throwing a golf disc stands at over 1,100 feet (335 meters).

The hard part is throwing the disc *accurately*. A ball thrown up in the air follows a relatively predictable, parabolic path, largely determined by the force of gravity acting on the sphere. It goes up, it comes down. Easy peasy. But unlike a spherical object, the trajectory of a flying disc is not something easily graphed and calculated in your Physics 101 class.

The force of gravity also applies to a spinning disc as it flies. However, the unique shape of the disc, and the rotational torque (spin) acting on it, make for a much more complex physics problem to solve. Disc golf is all about solving this physics problem in real time and in the real world.

As an object, such as a disc, flies through the air, it is constantly bumping into gas particles in the atmosphere, which gradually slow the disc down until it eventually comes to a stop on the ground. This is *wind, or air, resistance*. Also, the shape of a spinning disc thrown through the air generates *lift*, similar to the wings of an airplane. This means the air passing around the disc as it's flying exerts an upward force that keeps the disc aloft longer, which is why discs can

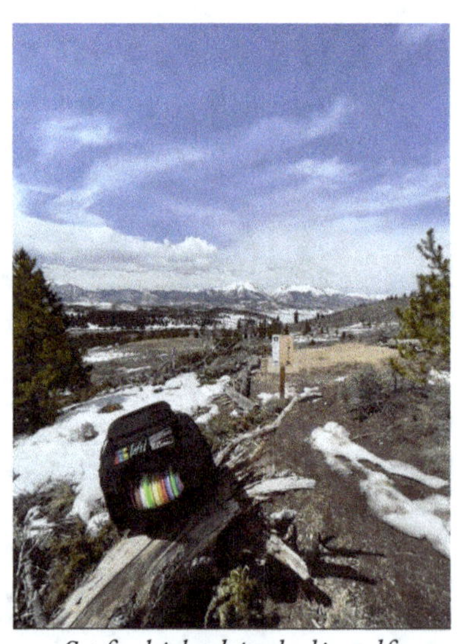

Set for high-altitude disc golf.

be thrown so much farther than balls. In summary, the air particles a disc encounters on its flight are responsible for both slowing down the disc due to air resistance and keeping the disc aloft due to lift. Fascinating!

Now here's where it gets really complicated. You see, flying discs do not travel in a straight line. A disc thrown through the air will actually travel in an S-shaped line. If thrown by a right-handed player, a disc will spin clockwise when viewed from above. When a disc leaves the golfer's hand, the clockwise spin will cause it to first start to drift to the right, then back to the left as the disc slows down, before finally landing on the ground. This tendency of flying discs to travel in an S-shaped line is termed *stability*.

Stability is the result of rotational torque and unequal air pressures generated on opposite sides of the disc. Think about the clockwise spinning disc described above. The left side of the disc (at the 9 o'clock position) is spinning *into* the wind, in the same vector as the trajectory of the disc. The right side of the disc (at the 3 o'clock position) is spinning *away* from the wind, in the opposite vector of the disc's flight. This results in a high-pressure system on the left side of the disc, and a low-pressure system on the right side. Higher air pressure on the left means greater lift on the left. The result of that unequal lift is a gradual drifting of the disc to the right as it flies. This is the first half of the S-shaped flight path caused by a disc's stability.

To understand the second half of stability, we need to introduce another concept called *gyroscopic precession*. This is another complicated piece of physics, but it's the same principle that allows helicopters to maneuver around in the air and keeps you from falling when riding a hoverboard. Gyroscopic precession says that if you apply a perpendicular force to a spinning object, that force will be seen 90° away in the direction of spin from where the force was applied. Imagine the disc as the face of a clock. If it's spinning clockwise, an upward force applied at the 12 o'clock position (the front of the disc) will be felt at the 3 o'clock position (the right side of the disc). Likewise, a downward force applied at the 7 o'clock position will cause a downward force at the 10 o'clock position.

Due to wind resistance, the disc will be moving at a slower velocity through the air and spinning at a slower rate. Slower speed through the air means less lift force acting on the disc, causing it to sink toward the ground. Instead of the front of the disc slicing straight through the air like it did when it first left the golfer's hand, the directional force of the air starts to push upward underneath the front of the disc. In other words, the disc is falling onto the air while it flies forward, and the air is now applying an upward force against the front of the disc.

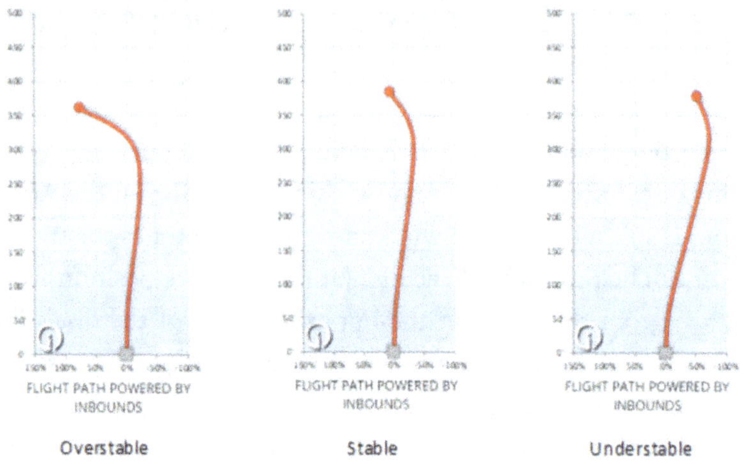

So, if our disc is spinning clockwise, and now there is an upward force applied at the 12 o'clock position, then according to gyroscopic precession, the disc should feel an upward force at the 3 o'clock position. This upward force on the right side of the disc causes it to drift back toward the left until it eventually slows down to the point of landing on the ground.

Okay, that was a lot, so let's put it all together! A golf disc is thrown by a right-handed player. The disc starts out flying through the air very fast and spinning at a high rate in a clockwise direction. The fast-spinning disc creates higher pressure on the left side than the right due to air resistance. This left-side pressure lifts and pushes the disc to the right as it's flying. The disc starts to slow down and begins to fall, resulting in an upward force of air against the front of the disc, at the 12 o'clock position. This upward-air force produces a gyroscopic force 90° away at the 3 o'clock position. The upward force on the right side of the disc causes it to move back toward the left while it continues to slow, and it eventually lands on the ground.

Now that we know how discs are supposed to fly and how the atmospheric forces determine a disc's flight, what changes should we expect to see when playing disc golf at high altitude?

At 9,000 feet (2,700 meters) elevation and higher, there are significantly fewer gas particles in the atmosphere for discs to bump into during flight. In other words, a disc will have less air resistance to deal with. That means it should fly faster and farther, right? Not necessarily.

Remember, the atmosphere not only slows the disc down due to air resistance, it also provides the lift that keeps the disc up in the air for so long. Fewer gas particles in the atmosphere also mean less lift force.

So, do discs fly longer, shorter, or the same distances at high altitude? The answer is, it depends. Again, flying discs are a much more complicated physics problem than an airborne baseball. Discs may fly longer or shorter distances at high altitude compared to sea level, but it depends on the type of disc, the player, and a whole host of other environmental factors, such as specific elevation, temperature, humidity, and the direction of the wind.

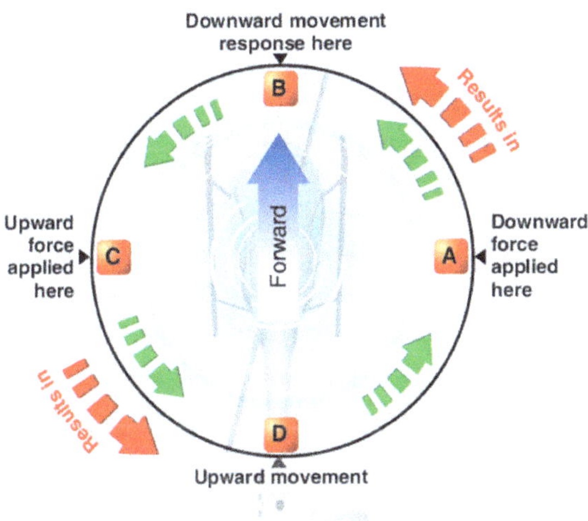

What we can say, however, is that discs do fly differently at altitude. The shape of the S-path a disc takes at high altitude will look different due to the reduced air density, and this can spell trouble for disc golfers who are expecting their discs to turn right when instead they turn left.

During the first half of the stability S-curve, the disc is normally pushed to the right due to the lift pressure created by air resistance. At high altitude, less air resistance means less lift pressure generated during this first half of the S-curve, so the disc doesn't move toward the right as much.

The second half of the S-curve is also different. As we said before, less atmosphere means less lift, so at high altitude, the disc will start to fall from its flight path sooner. That means the upward air force on the front of the disc that results when it starts to fall will also occur sooner in the disc's flight. Remember, this is the force that is felt by the disc 90° away on the right side of the disc that pushes the disc to the left for the final part of its flight path.

At high altitudes, discs drift less toward the right during the first half of the S-curve and begin the second half of the S-curve sooner along their flight path. The result is that discs fly not so much in an S-shaped path, but rather a J-shaped, or hook-shaped, path.

There you have it: high-altitude disc golf in a nutshell. It was initially very frustrating when I started playing in Summit County. The high altitude forces you to think about each hole and each shot differently than you might at sea level. The thin air changes the game dramatically, but that's what I love most about disc golf: it's a game that is virtually impossible to master, constantly challenges you, and can be enjoyed outside in the most beautiful and extreme environments. Pick out a disc at your local sporting goods store and give it a try.

Nonfreezing Cold Injury

An eighteen-year-old NorAm skier, NCAA Division I rugby player, and lover of the outdoors presented to our clinic complaining of cold, painful hands. She stated her hands always felt cold, with severe pain on colder days. Blood tests to rule out vascular disease were normal. What could be the cause of this?

In cold weather, the body works to keep essential organs functioning, but skin is not a priority. With exposure, blood vessels constrict to decrease blood flow to the skin. The metabolic demand of skin is low, so blood is shunted to more important organs, such as the heart and brain. Paradoxically, exposure to cooler temperatures, like those below 15° C (59° F), can cause cold-induced vasodilation. This allows blood to flow to the skin to help prevent more serious injury or frostbite. The vasodilation cycles in intervals of five to ten minutes.

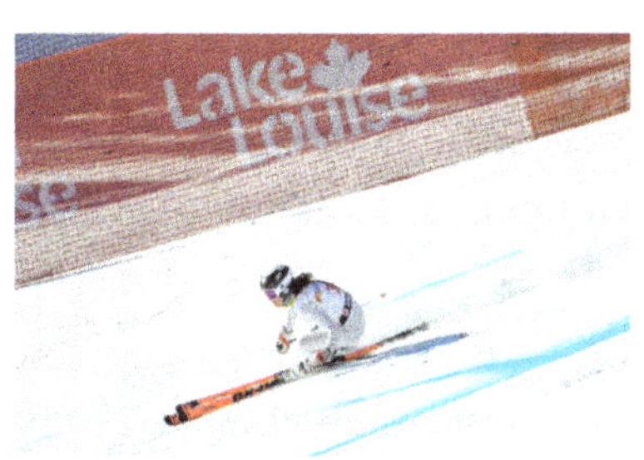

Jenna Sheldon, ski racing.

Nonfreezing cold injury (NFCI) occurs when tissues are damaged due to prolonged exposure to cold, but not freezing, temperatures. NFCI is due to exposure of the extremities, commonly hands and feet, to temperatures between 0°–15° C (32°–59° F). Current theory holds that NFCI is due to a combination of vascular and neural dysfunction. The skin experiences reduced blood flow with a neurological component also influencing the damage.

The Inuit, Sami people, and Nordic fishermen, indigenous to a cold environment, have a larger cold-induced vasodilation response and more rapid cycling, which may decrease their risk of NFCI. Is it possible that patients who develop NFCI have a smaller and slower cycling of their cold-induced vasodilation? Could this be the issue with our patient? Further research is needed to learn more about NFCI and find better ways to treat it.

We do know there are four stages of NFCI:

Stage 1: Loss of sensation, numbness, and clumsiness during the cold exposure. Usually painless unless rewarming is attempted.

Stage 2: Occurs during and after rewarming, following cold exposure. Skin can develop a mottled, pale, blue-like color. The area continues to feel cold and numb, with possible swelling lasting a few hours to several days.

Stage 3: Hyperemia. Affected area becomes red and painful. This begins suddenly and can last for several days to weeks.

Stage 4: Following hyperemia, affected areas appear normal but are hypersensitive to the cold. Areas may remain cold, even after short exposure. This stage can last for weeks to years.

Outdoor paddle sports like kayaking and canoeing put patients at the greatest risk due to continual exposure to cold, wet environments. It was thought that in order to have NFCI, one had to be exposed to environments that are both cold and wet. However, it has been shown this is not always the case. Like in our patient, exposure to cold alone can trigger the syndrome. Our eighteen-year-old patient is an avid skier and spends most of the winter on the mountain. It was also noted that she enjoys paddleboarding and kayaking, which were recognized as triggers for the hand pain. We were unable to determine exactly what caused our patient to develop this syndrome, but we do know it affects her life significantly.

We choose to live in the mountains because of the things we love to do. Whether it's hiking, biking, skiing, kayaking, paddleboarding, or the hundreds of other activities offered in this area, we are at risk of NFCI. Potential treatment for this syndrome with Iloprost, which can dilate blood vessels, is under investigation. Prevention is best, though.

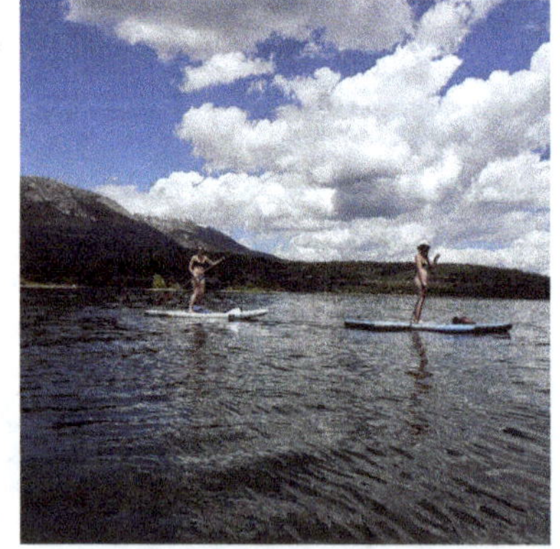

Stand up paddling Lake Dillon, Colorado.

The purpose of this book is to share information about staying healthy at high altitude, and sharing this information about the stages of NFCI with friends and family can help prevent this painful, debilitating condition.

REFERENCES

1. Nonfreezing cold water (trench foot) and warm water immersion injuries. UpToDate. https://www.uptodate.com/contents/nonfreezing-cold-water-trench-foot-and-warm-water-immersion-injuries. Accessed July 14, 2022.

2. Oakley B, Brown HL, Johnson N, Bainbridge C. Nonfreezing cold injury and cold intolerance in Paddlesport. Wilderness & Environmental Medicine. 2022;33(2):187-196. doi:10.1016/j.wem.2022.03.003.

**PART V
CHILDREN**

Can I Take My Child up a Fourteener?

There are over fifty "fourteeners"—mountains with an elevation of at least 14,000 feet (4,300 meters)—in Colorado. When summited, these majestic peaks afford their climbers spectacular views of the surrounding landscape. Being that many people within Colorado, as well as those who come to visit, are active, a question often voiced by parents is, "Can my child hike up a fourteener with me?" There is no straightforward answer to this question, and the simplest response is, it depends.

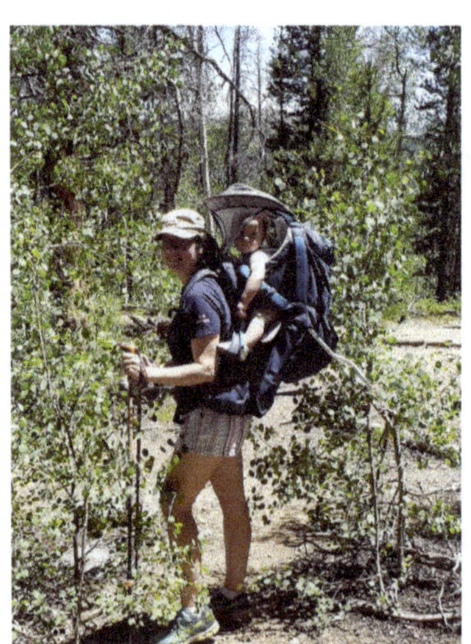

Copper Mountain residents Raquel and Victoria Santos, on the trail.

According to recent research, it appears children are largely similar to adults when it comes to adapting to higher elevations. Research examined children's short-term cardiorespiratory adaptation, incidence of acute mountain sickness, hypoxic ventilatory response, and maximal exercise capacity and found little variance between adults and children.[1]

When *can* you take your child up a fourteener? There are a multitude of factors that affect when and if a child is ready. For example, children develop and mature at different rates.

This means your eleven-year-old might be able to make the climb while another eleven-year-old may not. Additionally, some children grow up exposed to technical hikes and climbs, while others don't. Inexperienced children may find the hike is an exciting adventure or a big bore![4] If your child has an underlying condition, such as congenital heart disease, asthma, sickle cell anemia, upper respiratory infection, or ear infection, this can significantly increase the risk for high-altitude illnesses.[1]

Another factor is whether you live at altitude or are visiting from a lower elevation. Individuals traveling from a lower altitude are strongly encouraged to take some time to acclimate by spending a night or two at an intermediate altitude.

So, what's the bottom line? Since it isn't possible to place a concrete age on when it's okay for your child to climb a fourteener, it is ultimately up to you to know your child's limits and decide if such a challenging hike is right for you and for your child. The most important thing is to make sure everyone remains safe.

If you do decide to set out on the challenge of hiking up a fourteener, here is some advice to keep yourself and your child as safe as possible and ensure the hike is an enjoyable experience for all:[3]

Set out early. Summiting the peak by noon is recommended in order to avoid bad afternoon weather, such as thunderstorms and potential lightning strikes.

Start slow and easy. It's important for you to determine whether or not your child will be able to summit a fourteener. Start with easy hikes and build up over time so you have a good understanding of your child's abilities.

Know the weather forecast. Check the weather before you set out to prevent getting stuck in a storm.

Wear appropriate attire. It is important to layer since it can be colder on top of the mountain. Additionally, it is important to wear clothing that protects you from the elements (including the sun!).

Protect yourself from sun and wind. The sun can be very strong at altitude, so it's important to use sunscreen, proper clothing, and other measures to ensure your child is adequately protected from the sun. If you are carrying a baby in a backpack, have someone check that the child is well covered, and monitor the baby for exposure by feeling the temperature of the baby's cheeks and hands. Pernio, or chilblains, can develop when fat deposits under the cheeks are damaged.

Consider food and fluids. Bring adequate nutrition and hydration.

Be prepared to turn around. There are many things that could cause you to turn around ahead of time. It's important to accept in advance—and be okay with—the possibility that you might not summit the peak.

Be aware of high-altitude illness. It's imperative you know the symptoms of high-altitude illness and be prepared to turn around should your child exhibit any of them. Symptoms of high-altitude illness include fussiness or irritability, refusal to eat, lack of energy, nausea and/or vomiting, dizziness, and light-headedness.[4]

REFERENCES

1. Garlick, V., O'Connor, A., & Shubkin, C. D. (2017). High-altitude illness in the pediatric population: A review of the literature on prevention and treatment. Current Opinion in Pediatrics, doi:10.1097/MOP.0000000000000519.

2. How can I optimize my health at high altitude? (2016). Retrieved from http://www.altitudemedicine.org/optimizing-health-at-altitude.

3. Kirkland, E. (2015, May). Taking kids to new heights: Hiking Colorado's "14er" mountains. Retrieved from http://www.outdoorfamiliesonline.com/hiking-colorados-14er-mountains.

4. Provance, A.J. (n.d.). What age can my child start hiking fourteeners? Retrieved from https://www.childrenscolorado.org/conditions-and-advice/new-and-featured-articles/sports-safety/when-can-kids-start-hiking-fourteeners.

Your Baby or Child Is on Oxygen

*The following is from a handout distributed by **Christine Ebert-Santos, MD, MPS**, at Ebert Family Clinic in Frisco, Colorado.*

Living at high altitude is a challenge for our bodies. The amount of oxygen in the air we breathe decreases the higher we go, and since we all need oxygen to live, this can cause problems.

There are three times oxygen may be needed by children living at altitude:

1. During the newborn period
2. When a child has a respiratory illness, even a mild cold
3. During the first forty-eight hours after arriving (or returning) from sea level

When a baby takes their first breath, the higher oxygen level in the air sets off many changes in the heart, lungs, and blood vessels around the lungs that convert the child's respiratory system from transferring oxygen from the placenta to the lungs. Exposure to a low-oxygen environment during the first few weeks can interfere with the normal fall in blood vessel pressures in the lungs and the closing of vessels that had been shunting blood away from the lungs in the womb.

Hypoxia, the term for low oxygen in the blood, causes constriction, or narrowing, of the blood vessels in the lungs. This can lead to back pressure on the lungs and heart, causing fluid to leak into the air sacs in the short term, or hypertrophy of the heart muscle in the long term.

Normal oxygen saturation levels at 9,000 feet (2,700 meters) are 92%–93% but can be 89%–90% in healthy people. We start treating with oxygen below 89%, even though symptoms like trouble breathing, fast breathing, poor sleep, or poor color are unusual before the saturation level drops into the 70s.

It is important to understand that oxygen is prescribed by your doctor not only to treat symptoms of altitude sickness such as headache, vomiting, and trouble breathing, but also to prevent more severe symptoms from developing. A small percentage of patients with mildly low oxygen levels will suddenly, over a few hours, go into full-blown pulmonary edema, where their lungs fill with fluid, they have much more trouble breathing, and they turn blue. This is a life-threatening emergency.

HOW TO KEEP OXYGEN ON YOUR CHILD

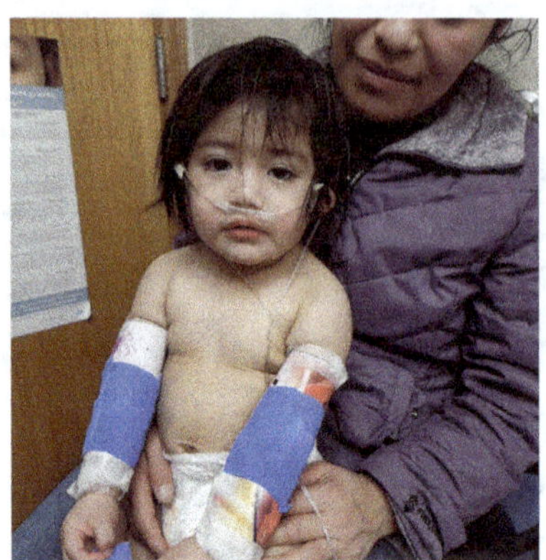

A pediatric patient surrenders to being on a nasal cannula for oxygen.

Rarely do babies or children with low oxygen levels at altitude show symptoms, but during illnesses both visiting and local children may need supplemental oxygen. When you arrive home with your child on oxygen, be sure and call the respiratory therapist at the phone number on the tank so they can come to your house and teach you about the equipment. There are excellent providers available to set up tanks and concentrators so you can be comfortable at home with family and not have to stay in the hospital.

Don't feel discouraged if your toddler or young child is fighting the oxygen at first. They will usually adjust and accept the cannula in about thirty minutes. Note that it would be a mistake to admit these children to the hospital just because they won't keep the nasal cannulas in their noses. Hospital guidelines make it difficult for nurses to implement adequate control measures over these feisty little ones.

At Ebert Family Clinic, we have found a very effective method: magazines. Tape a magazine around both of the child's arms so that they cannot bend their elbows to pull off the cannula. After thirty minutes of not being able to use their arms, most children will accept the oxygen and the restraints can be removed.

Don't panic if the oxygen cannula falls off during the night or the tank runs out. In babies and children, we are not worried about brain damage from lack of oxygen due to altitude. The problems caused by low oxygen saturations (usually between 78%–88%) seen at altitude develop over days, weeks, or years due to changes in the heart and lungs.

Altitude Kids Are Built Different: How Pediatric Patients Born at Altitude Adapt Biologically to the Hypoxic Environment

One of the phenomena I experienced while caring for pediatric patients in Summit County was the image of a child with an oxygen saturation of 83% who wasn't in any respiratory distress. This got me thinking: do adaptations in children exposed to chronic hypoxia at altitude prepare them to encounter an episode of acute hypoxia?

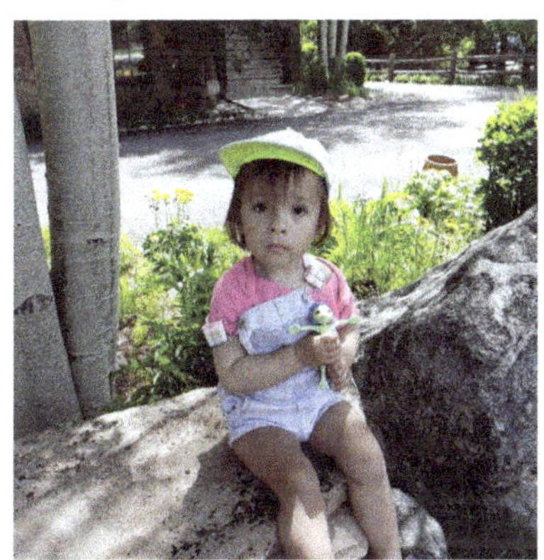

A young resident of Copper Mountain, Colorado, at 9,695 feet (2,955 meters).

Research shows that children permanently residing at high altitudes exhibit structural and functional variations to adapt to chronic hypoxia. For children living at altitudes greater than 3,000 meters (10,000 feet) above sea level since gametogenesis, the opportunities for phenotypic plasticity are particularly excellent.[1] Theorized and proven physiological differences in oxygen uptake, transport, systemic circulation, and consumption allow them to overcome the effects of chronic high-altitude hypoxia.

Visitors to the mountains experience the lower partial pressure of oxygen as less oxygen in the air. Increased respiratory effort is required to maintain the same oxygen levels as those children living at sea level. Children living at altitude have physiological increases in ventilation, lung compliance, and pulmonary diffusion, decreasing the need for augmented respiratory effort. Increases in lung compliance and tidal volume contribute to the effectiveness of oxygen exchange without requiring faster respirations. A study by Mortola, J.P. et al. showed lung compliance and tidal volume remained increased even while participants were on 100% supplemental oxygen. This suggests a permanent physiological adaptation in kids living at altitude.[2]

Resident high-altitude children are more efficient at delivering oxygen to their tissues. Pulmonary diffusion capacity, determined by the surface area available for diffusion, measures this improvement in oxygen delivery. Assuming all other anatomic variables are the same in highlanders and lowlanders,[2] this increased capacity can only be explained by an increase in the number and size of alveoli.[1] Researchers compared the lung volumes and chest dimensions of children exposed to chronic hypoxia at altitude since birth to those of children living at sea level, and found the dimensions of children residing at altitude were indeed greater.

The partial pressure of oxygen in blood is substantially lower. This decrease in arterial blood oxygen concentration associated with hypoxia encourages the kidneys to release erythropoietin, stimulating the production of erythrocytes, which contributes to an increased red blood cell and hemoglobin concentration in children living at altitude. The resulting increase in arterial oxygen saturation compensates for the lower availability of oxygen at altitude.[1]

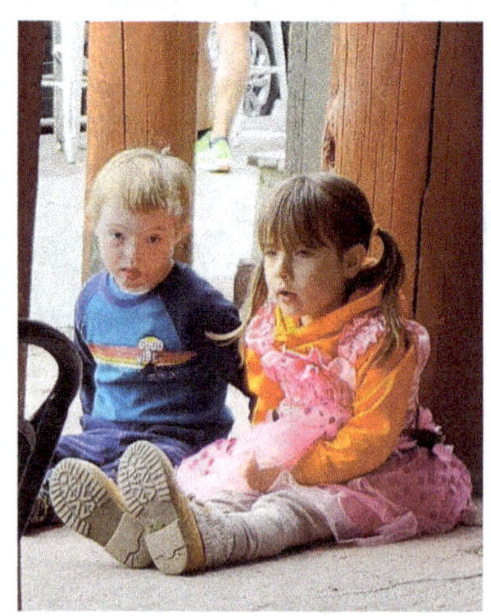

Kids in Summit County, Colorado.

Does chronic hypoxemia in this population result in decreased oxygen consumption? New research shows that the decrease in oxygen metabolism in newborns at altitude are reactions to acute stress and hypoxia, not an effect of chronic exposure to hypoxia.[1] The ability of children living at altitude to decrease ventilation during an episode of acute hypoxia is due to a decrease in tissue metabolism only during that event of respiratory stress.

These biological advantages do not come without consequences, however. Humans exposed to chronic hypoxia may develop elevated pressures in the lung blood vessels. Phenotypic, physiological changes in tidal volume and lung diffusion that improve oxygen uptake contribute to pulmonary hypertension. Compared to children who develop pulmonary hypertension unrelated to altitude, highland children often present with less-severe clinical pictures with fewer irreversible complications.[1]

Children born and residing at altitude offer a window into a world of medical phenomena unique to their hypoxic environment. Knowing about the physiological differences in this population leads to improved medical care.

REFERENCES

1. de Meer, K. et al. "Physical Adaptation of Children to Life at High Altitude." European Journal of Pediatrics, vol. 154, no. 4, Apr. 1995, pp. 263–72. Springer Link, https://doi.org/10.1007/BF01957359.

2. Mortola, J.P. et al. "Compliance of the Respiratory System in Infants Born at High Altitude." The American Review of Respiratory Disease, vol. 142, no. 1, July 1990, pp. 43–48. PubMed, https://doi.org/10.1164/ajrccm/142.1.43.

Mountain Kids are Smaller

How does living at high altitude affect the human body? It's a complicated question that researchers have been trying to answer for years.

It takes two things to grow: adequate nutrition and the body's ability to convert calories into energy. Observations over twenty-five years at the Ebert Family Clinic suggest that the decreased oxygen levels at altitude may interfere with optimal utilization of calories or decrease appetite and intake in small children.

After opening her pediatric clinic in Frisco, Colorado, in 2000, **Dr. Christine Ebert-Santos** noticed that children living at high altitude are smaller than average. Dr. Chris and **Meredith Caines Pollaro**, an occupational therapist with expertise in feeding and growth in children, organized a group for parents of underweight children but did not find any consistent abnormalities. After this, Dr. Chris decided that smaller growth might be a normal pattern for little ones at altitude. The children were otherwise healthy, with nutritional analysis showing adequate intake and no signs of endocrine or gastrointestinal problems.

Research on growth in children at altitude is sparse. So, in 2009, Dr. Chris recruited her daughter **Anicia Santos** to launch a detailed data analysis. Anicia worked with one of her math professors at the University of Colorado to convert the data into a unique growth chart for altitude that demonstrated the downward shift. Twice the number of infants and toddlers had weights below the third percentile of the World Health Organization growth charts than those at lower altitudes. Heights were also reduced. After years of gathering data, Dr. Chris and Anicia shared their findings with the help of **Logan Spector, PhD**, and graduate student **Aaron Clark**.

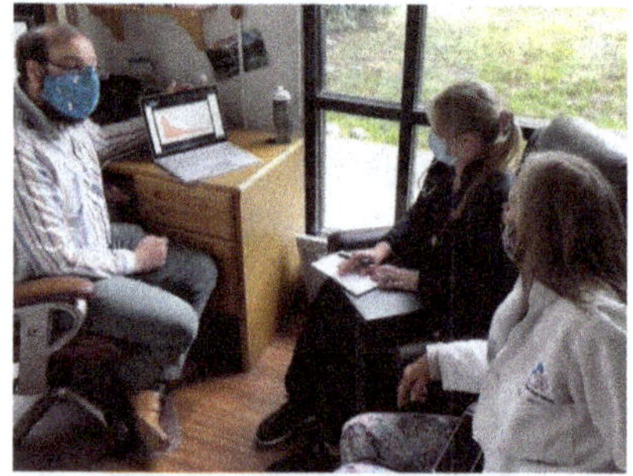

Graduate student Aaron Clark, reviewing high-altitude growth charts with PA student Laura Van Steyn and Dr. Christine Ebert-Santos.

Spector, chairman of the department of epidemiology at the University of Minnesota, was concerned about his two nieces who lived in Summit County and were not fitting into the "normal" growth pattern. This sparked his interest in Dr. Chris's research, and he was able to recruit Clark to take on the project.

In the first study of its kind in North America, the growth charts of 970 kids living in Colorado's high country were analyzed. With over 9,000 pieces of data, one thing was clear: from birth to eighteen months of age, children living at altitude weighed much less than the average child. Length was also considerably decreased, though the weight discrepancies were more drastic.

These findings were statistically significant. Using the generalized estimating equation (GEE), Clark was able to analyze the data in a non-linear way, which compensated for correlated data. Clark also created density graphs for both male and female children to depict these findings (see figures). When the graph line is fairly close to 1 on the y-axis, or a straight line across the top, this means there is little difference from the standard growth chart (ages 2–18). The farther away from 1 on the y-axis, the more significant difference there is compared to standard growth charts (ages 0–2). There is no denying that something is causing these high-altitude children to grow below the parameters set by studies on sea-level children.

The next logical question is, what are the effects of this smaller growth rate? Initial research shows that children at altitude are catching up on the growth curve by age two. There do not appear to be any long-lasting deficits from the initial smaller growth.

A study from Ladakh, India, also displays a correlation between children living at high altitude and smaller size. Another study shows lower birth weights at high altitude, specifically in Colorado, but it does not follow the growth patterns of the children over time.

From what this research shows, a unique growth chart for children living at high altitude would be helpful. This new chart would account for the variations in size seen at altitude. This could save thousands of dollars on unnecessary testing looking for underlying disease or endocrine deficiencies. It would also help lessen the anxiety parents feel when told their children have failure to thrive or are not being fed. Instead of being concerned when children fall low on the growth chart, they'll know that seeing smaller children at altitude is to be expected.

There is still much research to be done in this field, and hopefully, this study will serve as fuel for future studies.

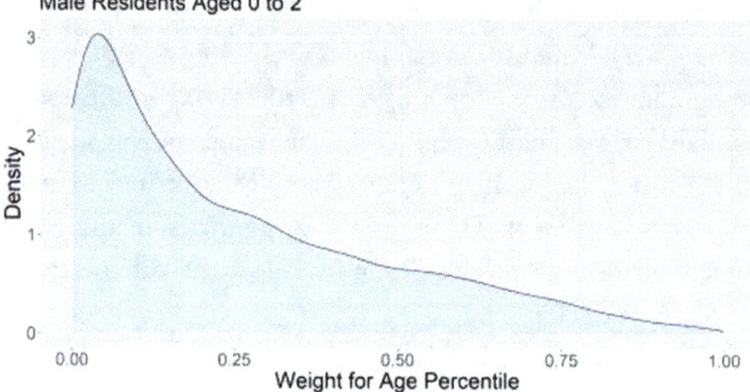

Density of Growth Percentiles of Weight for Age
Male Residents Aged 0 to 2

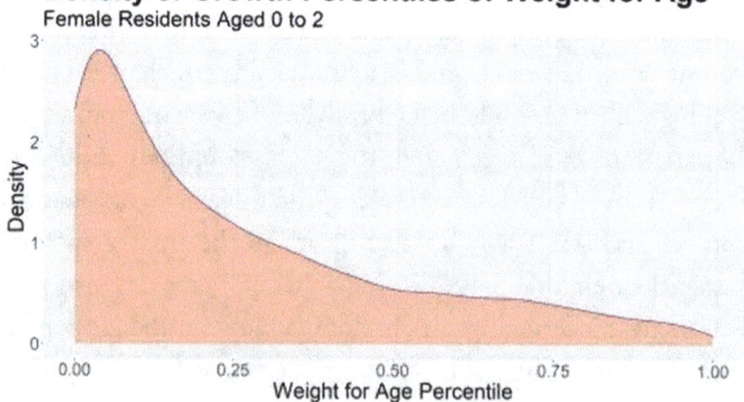

Density of Growth Percentiles of Weight for Age
Female Residents Aged 0 to 2

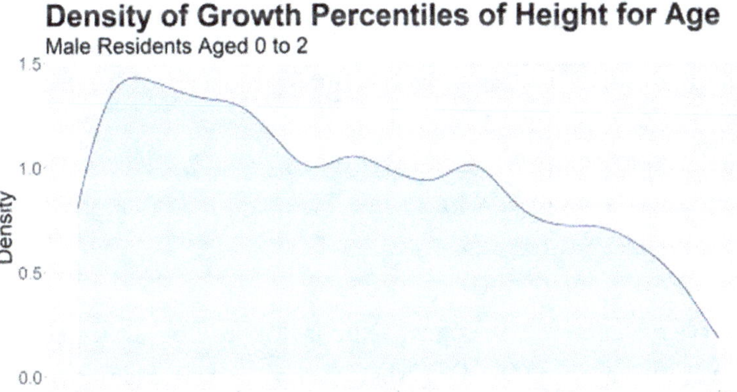

Density of Growth Percentiles of Height for Age
Male Residents Aged 0 to 2
1.5
1.0
0.5
0.0
Density
0.00
0.25
0.50
0.75
1.00
Height for Age Percentile

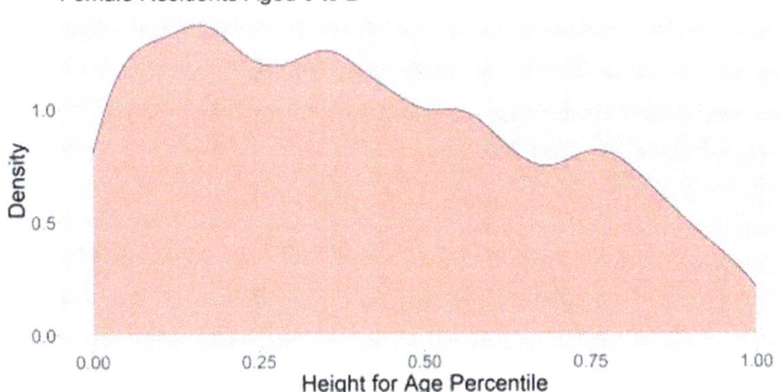

Density of Growth Percentiles of Height for Age
Female Residents Aged 0 to 2
1.0
0.5
0.0
Density
0.00
0.25
0.50
0.75
1.00
Height for Age Percentile

**PART VI
HEALTH & SAFETY**

How Do You Define a Good Night's Sleep?: An Introduction to the SleepImage Ring (Interview with Dr. Neale Lange)

Dr. Neale Lange is a leader in sleep medicine who started his medical training in South Africa and now practices pulmonary and sleep medicine for UCHealth in Denver.

Sleep plays a crucial role in cognitive behavior, and physical wellbeing is often taken for granted. As **Dr. Neale Lange** puts it, many people have been taught or trained to devalue sleep in an effort to maximize time awake to study, catch up on work, or complete other tasks.[1] However, research over the years has demonstrated that the toll sleep deprivation takes on the body is significant. Sleep deprivation can lead to impairment in memory, cognition, and emotion, as well as chronic medical conditions such as diabetes, heart disease, and cancer.[2] It is also thought that sleep deprivation and hypoxemia are associated with white matter disease in the brain and that deep, slow-wave sleep is what fixes it.[4]

Dr. Lange states that sleeping at altitude carries its own risks. There is less oxygen in the air, causing overall poor sleep quality, frequent arousals, marked nocturnal hypoxia, and periodic breathing. Additionally, sleeping at altitude can negatively impact our sleep architecture, increasing the amount of light sleep and decreasing the amount of deep, slow-wave and REM sleep, which play a key role in memory creation and retention, emotional control, and personal behavior.[3]

In hopes of defining a person's sleep at altitude, Dr. Lange started a sleep lab in Summit County at St. Anthony Summit Hospital, which, as he put it, "opened a can of worms" when he saw how sick and complicated patients' sleep apnea symptoms were. Time and time again, he saw that when patients who were struggling with sleep apnea were given two liters of supplemental oxygen by nasal cannula, the apnea improved. Additionally, those patients with sleep apnea who descended 4,000 feet (1,219 meters) to Denver had improved saturations but may still have had sleep apnea. His facility study included baseline tests at two hours without oxygen and then two hours with oxygen while a person slept. He found that although the apnea improved in many, sleep quality did not always get better.

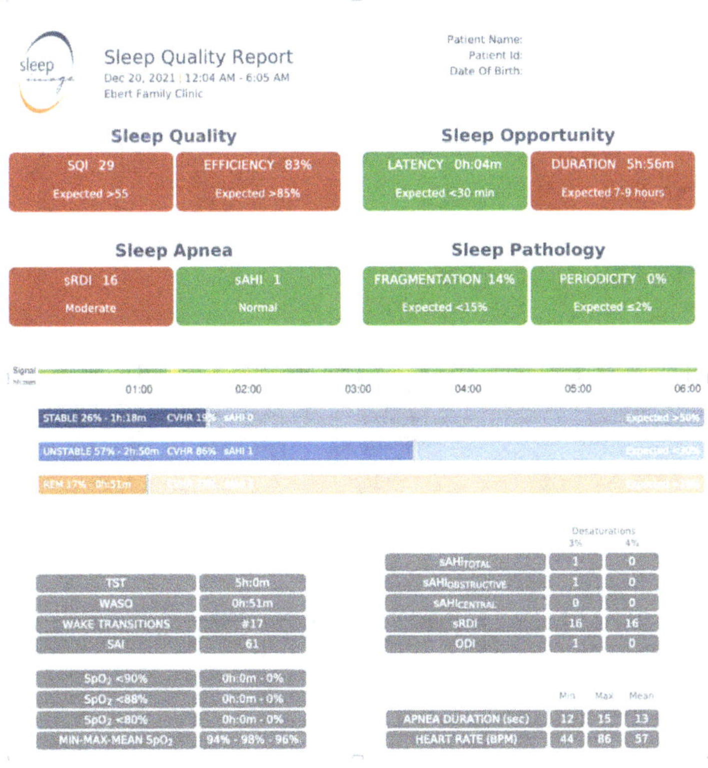

Sleep quality report.

This left him with the question of: how do we measure "good sleep"? As he states, it's not that simple. Though the obvious answer may be to turn to medications to determine good sleep, this can be misleading. Medications have an amnestic effect on people, so if their memories are blank when they wake up in the morning, they feel they've had a good night's rest. In reality, this is subjective. The true data collected during sleep is objective, so to answer his question of measuring sleep, he turns to a tool of cardiopulmonary coupling (CPC): the **SleepImage Ring**, which looks like an Apple Watch and is worn around a patient's finger throughout the night. Using Bluetooth technology, data is collected and transferred through a smartphone for analysis, providing the patient with a vast amount of data about their sleep.

The SleepImage System is the only FDA-approved medical-grade technology on the market with the simplicity of a consumer device for use in both children and adults. It is intended for use by a healthcare professional to establish a patient's sleep quality and aid in evaluation and clinical diagnosis of sleep disorders and sleep-disordered breathing, or SDB.

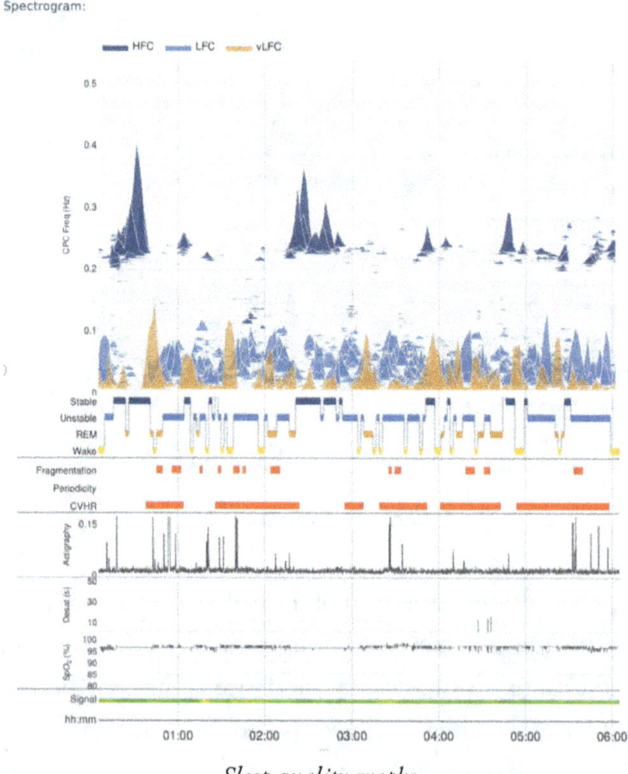

Sleep quality graphs.

It uses CPC technology, which is "based on calculations and spectral analysis of cardiovascular and respiratory data" collected during sleep, with a "normal sinus rhythm ECG or PLETH (plethysmogram from a PPG sensor) signal as the only input requirement."

The output metrics from the SleepImage System include "sleep duration (SD), total sleep time (TST), wake after sleep onset (WASO), and sleep quality (SQI). Measurements related to apnea or sleep-disordered breathing include an Oxygen Desaturation Index (ODI), Apnea-Hypopnea Index (sAHI), Respiratory Disturbance Index (sRDI), Central Sleep Apnea Index, and the Sleep Apnea Indicator (SAI) that is derived from Cyclic Variation in Heart Rate (CVHR).[6] With a PLETH signal including saturations, the SDB data conforms with the American Academy of Sleep Medicine AHI scoring and severity definitions."

Additionally, we can determine how long a patient spends in various sleep stages, including stable, unstable, and REM sleep, and determine apnea events and autonomic nervous system activity. The data is generated and presented on the SleepImage Quality Report (shown in the graphics). The ring and report are designed to allow individualized, precise sleep medicine. "The devil is in the details," says Dr. Lange, referring to the vast amount of information that can be analyzed from just one night of sleep.

Currently, the gold standard of monitoring and diagnosing sleep disorders is polysomnography, also known as a sleep study, which records certain body functions as patients sleep to determine brain activity, oxygen, heart rate, breathing, as well as eye and leg movements.[5] It can also detect types of sleep apnea. One disadvantage, however, is that since it is typically conducted during an overnight stay in a hospital or sleep center, it takes people out of their natural sleeping environments. The cost, time waiting for appointments, and inconvenience deter many from participating.

Dr. Lange explains that due to the ease of wearing the device over multiple nights (compared to spending one night in a sleep lab for a study), the SleepImage Ring can change the way we look at our sleep and provide better insight into our sleep on a greater scale. A study done on 65,000 users found added benefit to multi-night testing compared to single-night testing. Sleep apnea has been shown to vary from night to night, indicating that single-night testing potentially misclassifies 20% of people.[7] This device provides the ease of multi-night testing for patients, which is a significant advantage, and increases accurate diagnosis of sleep-disordered breathing. To Dr. Lange, "it is about individualized patient care" and evaluating "the person sitting in front of [him]" that makes this device so valuable. Dr. Lange states that "living at altitude is a particular challenge, and if people are thinking ahead," then instead of wondering, "How long do I want to live at altitude?" they will ask, "How can I invest in brain wellness?"

In summary, sleep deprivation, especially at altitude, is a problem people should not overlook. At Ebert Family Clinic in Frisco, Colorado, every patient is asked, "How did you (or your child) sleep last night?" Now, with the SleepImage Ring, we can objectively evaluate our patients' sleep, aiding in the diagnosis and management of various conditions. We have also found that most patients have an improvement of over 60% in sleep apnea using oxygen by nasal cannula alone, without CPAP. "Doc, that's the best I've slept since I got here," many people say after their first night on oxygen.

Dr. Lange and Dr. Ebert-Santos continue to study the effects of high altitude on sleep and present their findings at conferences. They want patients, providers, and scientists to know that a simple intervention can improve your brain, heart, and body while you enjoy life in the mountains.

REFERENCES

1. South African Dental Association. (2021, November 25). The sleep disorder spectrum: Mouth breathing to Osa - Dr Neale Lange (WEB126). YouTube. Retrieved December 5, 2021, from https://www.youtube.com/watch?v=agZruGNfFNI.

2. Irish, L. A., Kline, C. E., Gunn, H. E., Buysse, D. J., & Hall, M. H. (2015). The role of sleep hygiene in promoting public health: A review of empirical evidence. Sleep medicine reviews, 22, 23–36. https://doi.org/10.1016/j.smrv.2014.10.001.

3. Wickramasinghe, H., & Anholm, J. D. (1999). Sleep and Breathing at High Altitude. Sleep & breathing = Schlaf & Atmung, 3(3), 89–102. https://doi.org/10.1007/s11325-999-0089-1.

4. Voldsbekk, I., Groote, I., Zak, N., Roelfs, D., Geier, O., Due-Tønnessen, P., Løkken, L. L., Strømstad, M., Blakstvedt, T. Y., Kuiper, Y. S., Elvsåshagen, T., Westlye, L. T., Bjørnerud, A., & Maximov, I. I. (2021). Sleep and sleep deprivation differentially alter white matter microstructure: A mixed model design utilizing advanced diffusion modelling. NeuroImage, 226, 117540. https://doi.org/10.1016/j.neuroimage.2020.117540.

5. Mayo Foundation for Medical Education and Research. (2020, December 1). Polysomnography (Sleep Study). Mayo Clinic. Retrieved December 25, 2021, from https://www.mayoclinic.org/tests-procedures/polysomnography/about/pac-20394877#:~:text=Polysomnography%2C%20also%20called%20a%20sleep,leg%20movements%20during%20the%20study.

6. MyCardio LLC. (2021, November 24). Introduction to sleepimage®. Retrieved December 10, 2021, from https://sleepimage.com/wp-content/uploads/Introduction-to-SleepImage.pdf.

7. Lechat, B., Naik, G., Reynolds, A., Aishah, A., Scott, H., Loffler, K. A., Vakulin, A., Escourrou, P., McEvoy, R. D., Adams, R. J., Catcheside, P. G., & Eckert, D. J. (2021). Multi-night Prevalence, Variability, and Diagnostic Misclassification of Obstructive Sleep Apnea. American journal of respiratory and critical care medicine, 10.1164/rccm.202107-1761OC. Advance online publication. https://doi.org/10.1164/rccm.202107-1761OC.

HAST: The High-Altitude Simulation Test

Maybe you're planning to ski or hike a fourteener. Or taking a leap of faith and moving out of the city and into the mountains. Maybe you just spent ten days in the hospital with rib fractures and are now anxious to return home to 9,000 feet (2,700 meters) of elevation. You might be worried about how you will feel on that incredible work retreat to a beautiful mountain sanctuary due to apprehension about your chronic obstructive pulmonary disease (COPD). Or maybe you're about to take a flight in a pressurized airplane cabin.

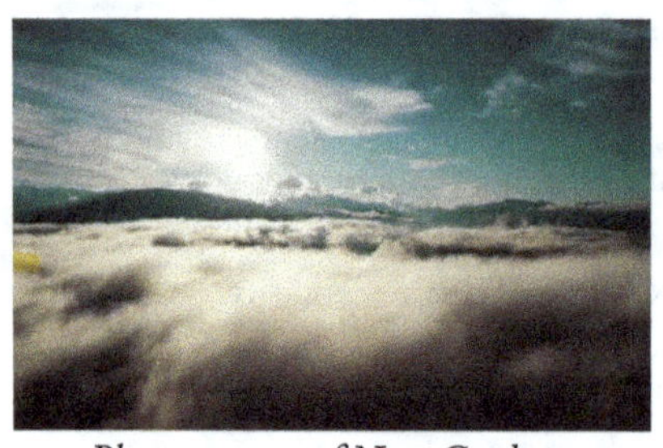

Photo courtesy of Nate Cordero.

Wouldn't it be nice to know how you'll respond to altitude prior to reaching your destination, so you can be better prepared?

That's exactly what the **high-altitude simulation test**, or **HAST**, is for. This test can simulate 8,000 feet (2,438 meters) of elevation in the safety of a doctor's office at a lower elevation. A HAST is a diagnostic test that can effectively calculate an individual's supplemental oxygen needs prior to traveling to high altitude. The California Thoracic Society recommends a HAST for individuals diagnosed with severe airway disease, cystic fibrosis, neuromuscular disease, or kyphoscoliosis; individuals who have been hospitalized for acute respiratory illness within the last six weeks; or individuals with previous air travel intolerance, COPD, or cerebral vascular disease prior to traveling to altitude (Corby-DeMaagd, 2020).

The HAST is performed by obtaining a patient's blood pressure, heart rate/rhythm, and oxygen saturation at baseline. Once baseline vitals are complete, the patient is monitored while breathing in a mixture of gases containing approximately 15.1% oxygen, simulating the FiO2 at an elevation of 8,000 feet (2,438 meters). A patient's oxygen saturation levels can be recorded by an arterial line (large IV in the wrist) monitoring the patient's arterial blood gases, or by an oxygen monitor attached to the patient's finger or nasal cannula. This allows the physician to screen for hypoxia, arrhythmias, or other significant symptoms. If the patient becomes symptomatic, oxygen levels are reassessed while providing supplemental oxygen to identify exactly how much oxygen would be needed to keep the patient comfortable at a higher altitude. This test, on average, takes two hours to complete (Corby-DeMaagd, 2020).

According to Mark Fleming, supervisor of Pulmonary Physiology Services at National Jewish Health in Denver, Colorado, for an individual to receive a HAST they would need a referral from a provider. National Jewish Health is one of the few facilities in the nation that provides this service. Most people who request this test in the state of Colorado are those interested in relocating to the mountains, people who are planning high-altitude vacations and are currently on supplemental oxygen, patients with histories of pulmonary embolism or lung resections, and pilots who have had recent ailments and need work clearance prior to being exposed to airplane cabin pressure. Fleming states they are also anticipating an increase in demand for high-altitude simulation testing for patients who have recovered from COVID-19.

There may be a vulnerable population that is not receiving the benefit of this test, such as newborn babies who are delivered at 5,000 feet (1,500 meters) and must return home to 8,500 feet (2,600 meters) or people who have experienced chest trauma and must return home to altitude. In our experience, many people who have had invasive surgeries that involve the lungs, chest, spine, or abdomen require oxygen at home post op. These are all individuals who would benefit from knowing whether they will need oxygen once they return to elevation.

High-Altitude Cerebral Edema (HACE) and Metabolism at Altitude: Can Nutrition Help?

My friend and I decided to go camping in an area close to Silverthorne, Colorado (9,035 feet, or 2,754 meters), above tree line at around 11,000 feet (3,352 meters). Both of us were endurance athletes and had done camping trips at altitude many times without complications. We considered ourselves in great shape and ready for any adventure.

We departed from our home in Fort Collins (5,003 feet, or 1,525 meters) in the morning and arrived at the trailhead before noon. We were well prepared, well hydrated, and had plenty of nutrition in our over forty–pound (18–kilogram) backpacks in preparation for the seven-mile (11.3-kilometer) hike to our destination. We built our camp and went to bed. Both of us had mild edema to our extremities, but nothing that we were worried about as we had experienced these symptoms on multiple hikes to higher elevations in the past.

We spent the next day hiking above tree line, staying hydrated and fueling with high-quality calories. We knew it was important to eat even when we didn't feel like it—a lesson we had learned when we both experienced weight loss of about five to ten pounds (2–4 kilograms) per week when camping and hiking above 10,000 feet (3,000 meters).

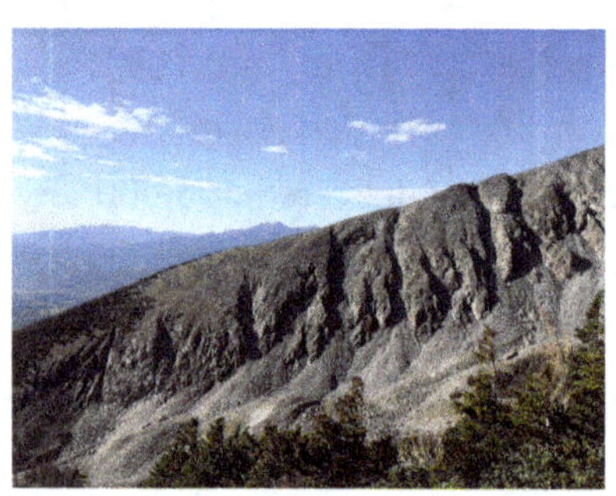

View from the summit of Mt. Shavano, a fourteener above Buena Vista, Colorado.

The next day, we did a seven-mile (11.3-kilometer) exploratory hike along the ridgeline at 11,000 feet (3,352 meters). We had just returned to camp when my partner first mentioned a mild pounding headache. He drank more fluids, had dinner, and went to bed.

I woke up around midnight when my partner scrambled out of the tent. He vomited once and crawled back inside. But something else seemed off: he didn't zip the tent door shut when he returned. Mumbling that his head was hurting, he kept his head elevated as it relieved the pain to some degree. A few hours later, he vomited again.

The next morning, he was still complaining of a pounding headache, so I proposed packing up camp and hiking back down the mountain. He refused, saying he wanted to hike some more. I left the tent site first and walked a few steps. When I turned around, he was sitting down, staring at the ground. Now I really started to get worried. My friend was an amazing endurance athlete with a never-ending hunger for adventure. This was not like him.

I decided to pack up the tent whether he liked it or not. We needed to get off the mountain before his condition worsened.

After many attempts, I was finally able to convince him to come with me and we started our descent. Because his coordination was slightly limited, we walked slowly down to 9,000 feet (2,743 meters). After that, his coordination started to improve; he was walking faster and communicating more. By the time we got back to our car, he was his normal self again. However, he still had a lingering headache.

The effects of altitude on his body were very surprising. He demonstrated some classic symptoms of what the high-altitude medical community refers to as **high-altitude cerebral edema** (**HACE**): headache, vomiting, confusion, and ataxia (loss of control of body movement). The experience was unexpected and scary. Cell phone reception was very limited in the backcountry, and if his condition had worsened, this trip could have ended in a very bad situation. The confusion and poor judgement manifesting during an episode of HACE has led to one hiker walking off a cliff.

Early suspicion of possible altitude-related conditions and good planning to maintain adequate calories are vital.

I recently had a conversation with an avid outdoorsman who calls Fort Collins home. He said he consistently experiences unwanted weight reduction of around five to ten pounds (2–4 kilograms) in body weight per week when living in the backcountry at elevations above 9,000 feet (2,743 meters).

Is this weight loss related to increased activity without adjusting calorie intake? Could this weight loss be related to exposure to higher elevation and possible changes in metabolism? How can one keep track of calorie cost and anticipate the inevitable stress on the body at altitude?

COMPARE YOUR ACTIVITY LEVEL

A GPS or even a pedometer can help measure and compare activity level. An increase in miles or steps compared to baseline may require caloric adjustment. In order to prevent weight loss, calorie input should equal calorie expenditure. It is important to take into consideration that hiking in the mountains usually requires a high level of physical performance due to uneven walking surfaces and the gain and loss in elevation, resulting in increased muscle recruitment.

INCREASED BASAL METABOLIC RATE (BMR)

According to Dünnwald et al. (2019), exposure to higher altitude increases BMR initially as the body is adapting to the hypoxic environment. The study concluded that increased sympathetic activity and hypoxia may be responsible for the increase in BMR. Involuntary shivering, due to more extreme exposure to elements such as cold, wind, rain, and snow, may also contribute to an increase in calorie expenditure and should be considered when preparing for the backcountry.

DECREASE IN APPETITE

Another factor contributing to possible weight loss may be related to a lack of appetite. Some researchers believe there may be a correlation between a change in appetite-stimulating hormones at altitude. A study by Shukla et al. (2005) found a decrease in total levels of the appetite-stimulating hormone ghrelin, peptide YY, glucagon-like peptide-1, and leptin at initial exposure to altitude. Pre-packaging and scheduling meals while hiking at altitude may aid in the prevention of weight loss during backcountry activities.

MUSCLE ATROPHY

Chaudhary et al. (2012) propose that changes in protein turnover in hypoxic environments may be related to muscle wasting, including a decrease in protein synthesis and an increase in protein degradation. To minimize muscle atrophy, it is important to consume high-protein foods frequently. Amino acids may also aid in protein synthesis. Packing snacks with high nutritional value can prevent weight loss. Nutrition labels on food items are a great way to identify optimal snacks.

Hiking in the backcountry on a multi-day trip requires preparation. I choose high-calorie foods that taste good, are light to pack, and have minimal waste. I make breakfast and dehydrated meals at home and put them into individual bags that only require me to add water. Making your own dehydrated meals allows you to avoid unnecessary additives. I supplement throughout the day with high-calorie snacks. If I have room in my pack, I also add what I call "novelty" backcountry foods, such as cheese and wine. It's important to splurge every once in a while, even if you live in a tent.

GREAT FOODS FOR THE BACKCOUNTRY

Butter or coconut-oil coffee. Many companies make pre-packaged individual coffees. One cup of butter coffee is around 200 calories.

Perfect Bars. One bar has around 300 calories and 17 grams of protein.

ProBars. One bar has 390 calories. They are light to pack and taste great.

Nuts and seeds. Easy to pack and a great source of healthy fats, calories, and protein.

Jerky. We make our own elk jerky. It's a great snack throughout the day with healthy protein and added salt.

Apples. It is difficult to get fresh fruit in the backcountry. Apples are easy to pack, last for a long time, and provide vitamins and fiber.

Dehydrated fruits and vegetables. Great addition to oatmeal in the morning and your dinner at night. Dehydrated fruits and vegetables are easy to make at home and very light to pack, and you can rehydrate them in the backcountry.

Oatmeal with protein powder. We pre-package oatmeal with dehydrated fruit and a scoop of our favorite protein powder in individual bags. Just add water and you have a fantastic-tasting and calorie-rich breakfast.

Every backcountry excursion should be well planned, and it is always better to be overprepared. It's crucial to be knowledgeable about what foods need to be consumed, and when, in order to prevent negative outcomes. Know the distances and elevation changes on your trip, prepare for changes in weather, plan out your calories for every meal on every day, and make a schedule to prevent complications related to nutrition.

Most importantly: enjoy the beauty of the high-elevation backcountry!

REFERENCES

1. Chaudhary, P., Suryakumar, G., Prasad, R., Singh, S.N., Ali, S., Ilavazhagan, G. (2012). Chronic hypobaric hypoxia mediated skeletal muscle atrophy: role of ubiquitin–proteasome pathway and calpains. Retrieved from: https://link.springer.com/article/10.1007%2Fs11010-011-1210-x.

2. Dünnwald, T., Gatterer, H., Faulhaber, M., Arvandi, M., Schobersberger, W. (2019). Body Composition and Body Weight Changes at Different Altitude Levels: A Systematic Review and Meta-Analysis. Retrieved from: https://www.frontiersin.org/articles/10.3389/fphys.2019.00430/full.

3. Shukla, V., Singh, S.N., Vats P., Singh, V.K. , Singh, S.B., Banerjee, P.K. (2005). Ghrelin and leptin levels of sojourners and acclimatized lowlanders at high altitude. Retrieved from: https://www.ncbi.nlm.nih.gov/pubmed/16117183.

Trouble Breathing at Altitude

She died on the Breckenridge bike path clutching her inhaler, I heard. For years I was reminded by a memorial along the path. Then a man called last week saying he was selling his house located at 10,500 feet (3,200 meters) because his trouble breathing interfered with skiing and rock climbing. "I use my inhaler fifty times a day," he told me. "The doctor said I have asthma."

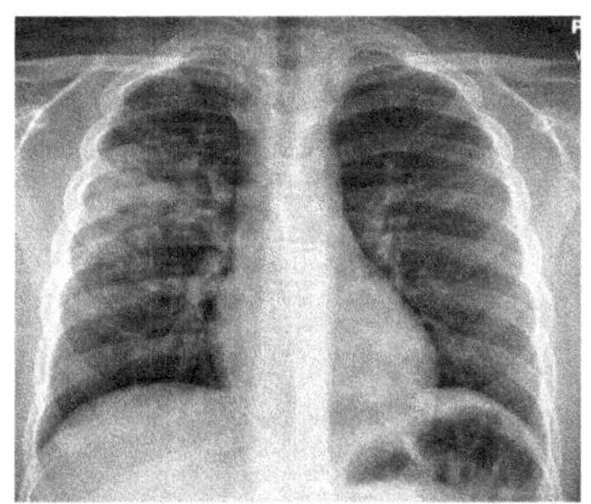

X-ray of patient with HAPE.

Recently, doctors in Summit County have started to question whether some people living at high altitude may have another cause of breathing problems, such as **high-altitude pulmonary edema (HAPE)** or **pulmonary hypertension**.

I frequently see children in my office with respiratory illnesses and low oxygen, with readings in the 80s or below. They are not leaning forward, gasping for air, and using their rib muscles to breathe like a person with an asthma attack severe enough to cause low oxygen. The stethoscope isn't picking up any wheezing. We usually give a trial of albuterol, since the medicine has minimal side effects and asthma is a common condition, but it rarely makes a big difference. We also test peak flows on patients over five to try and measure airway resistance seen in asthmatics. Then we send them home on oxygen, the treatment for HAPE, and they get better.

Many of the families whose children need oxygen during illnesses are evaluated by lung specialists at Colorado Children's Hospital or National Jewish Health. They are all told they have asthma and are treated with inhaled steroids and albuterol. Pulmonary testing in the older children suggests reversible airway disease in about half. Recently, a pulmonologist told us he didn't believe the child had HAPE and requested a chest X-ray at the time of any future episode.

Fulminant cases of HAPE do show dramatic changes in the X-rays, such as a recent case of a six-year-old who returned from sea level, whose oxygen dropped into the 40s overnight. Patients with milder illnesses often have clear lungs. The chest X-rays will not be abnormal until a day or two later. I rarely order X-rays to make a diagnosis.

Over two decades of experience treating hypoxic children in the mountains has convinced me they're usually experiencing a form of HAPE, with a small percentage also having underlying pneumonia or asthma. Children with only pneumonia are not hypoxic, and children with asthma are not hypoxic after being treated with bronchodilator therapy.

Altitude as Asthma Treatment

*Can **high-altitude climate therapy (HACT)** result in long-term benefits for adults with severe asthma?*

How much do you know about asthma? Have you ever considered that the air we breathe every day is often filled with environmental triggers that worsen asthma symptoms, making it more difficult for asthmatics to breathe? Do you realize that at elevation, many of those environmental triggers like air pollution and pollen are gone? The rumors are true: mountain air really is better, and residents at altitude are truly lucky to be breathing in fresh, clean, crisp mountain air on a daily basis.

Based on data collected by the Global Initiative for Asthma (GINA), as of 2004 it was estimated that 300 million people of all ages worldwide suffer from asthma. That number is projected to increase to 400 million by 2025. In 2010, the CDC documented that 1.8 million people in the United States alone visited the emergency department for asthma-related care, and of that number, at least one-third had to be hospitalized for severe symptoms.

Asthma is characterized by: 1) chronic airway inflammation, 2) intermittent and reversible airway obstruction, and 3) bronchial hyperresponsiveness (the tendency of airways to narrow in response to a variety of triggers in the air that have little effect on people with no respiratory disease). Patients with asthma often complain of intermittent cough, shortness of breath (or difficulty breathing), and wheezing. This classic presentation is often worsened by a variety of triggers, including allergens, pollutants, tobacco, cockroaches, pollen, mold, stress, upper respiratory infections, weather, and exercise. Symptoms are alleviated with bronchodilator medications, which act to open the airways, making breathing easier.

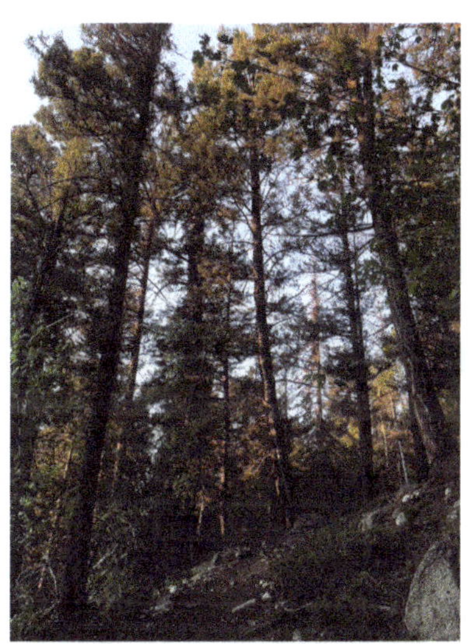

"Shinrinyoku" (森林浴) is the Japanese word for spending time in nature, literally meaning "deep forest bathing." It is believed the body exchanges and balances its ions with the ions present in the forest.

Asthma is conventionally treated in a stepwise fashion, meaning treatment escalates with increasing severity of symptoms. Patients who suffer from severe asthma on a daily and nightly basis are often on multiple medications in an attempt to control their symptoms. These usually include an inhaled corticosteroid medication, a long-acting beta-2 agonist. Some start oral steroids and others require biologic or immune modulating agents. Patients that fall into this category often suffer decreased quality of life, require multiple doctor or emergency room visits, and have difficulty controlling their symptoms on a regular basis.

Recently, researchers have been investigating different avenues to provide relief for patients suffering from severe asthma symptoms. Studies published on HACT show positive outcomes for adults with severe asthma that are refractory to conventional treatment.

An article published in 2018 in the *European Journal of Allergy and*

Clinical Immunology examined a study that was conducted to determine whether HACT resulted in long-term benefits for asthmatics even after returning to sea level. Patients included in this study had to fall into the category of adults with severe uncontrolled asthma symptoms despite conventional treatment methods. These patients were enrolled in a twelve-week, multi-disciplinary treatment program with environmental trigger avoidance in an alpine climate, at an altitude greater than 1,500 meters (4,921 feet). After the conclusion of the program, patients were followed for one year, with repeat evaluations every three months, to assess the long-term effects of this therapy on their asthma symptoms.

This is the first study to show a decrease in exacerbations and improvement in asthma control for up to twelve months, as measured by the number of asthma attacks, hospitalizations, and oral corticosteroid use before and after HACT treatment. The study showed a decrease in all three categories, which correlates to a positive outcome following this treatment.

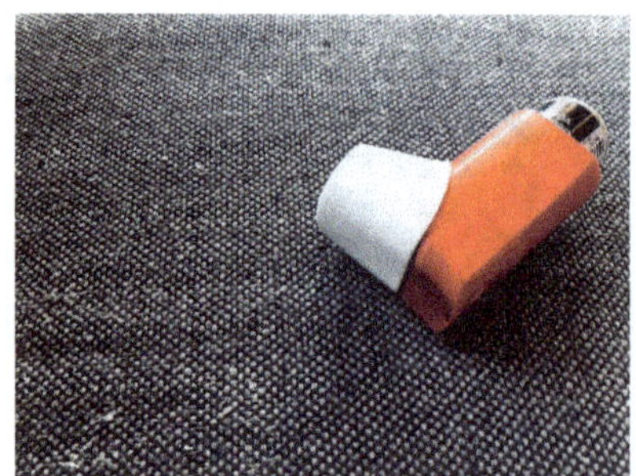

Albuterol inhaler for treatment of asthma.

While trigger avoidance has always been an important aspect of the conventional asthma treatment regimen, it is amazing to see how patients benefit when this is carried out effectively. It is hypothesized that allergens work to continually stimulate and maintain the airway inflammation in asthmatics. When these triggers are removed for a sufficient amount of time, the bronchioles have a chance to recover and decrease the process of ongoing inflammation.

Another proposed mechanism by which this treatment is effective is the decrease in air viscosity at altitude, which benefits the patient by decreasing the thickness of airway mucosa and may even reverse airway modeling. This makes breathing easier for patients and acts to decrease asthma symptoms.

So who can benefit from this treatment? Are all asthmatics created equal?

Scientists and clinicians alike have identified three different groups of asthma patients: those with 1) severe atopic asthma, 2) persistent eosinophilic asthma, and 3) asthma associated with morbid obesity. While classically, these different patient populations respond differently to asthma treatments, it has been found in another study, "Predictors of Benefit From High-Altitude Climate Therapy," that HACT improves the quality of life and respiratory function in all patients suffering from severe asthma symptoms. This study sought to investigate whether different factors such as age, blood eosinophils (a type of white blood cell), and degree of asthma control prior to admission could predict how much a patient would benefit from high-altitude climate therapy. While this study made strides in the right direction, it was determined that further patient characterization is required to clearly identify which patients will benefit the most from HACT.

Finally, in a systematic review and meta-analysis on HACT, it was found that patients experience a statistically significant improvement in lung function following this treatment modality.

Among some of the questions still being evaluated: What is the optimal altitude and duration of treatment that sees the greatest benefit? Which patients will experience the most improvement from this treatment? How does this treatment method compare financially with others, considering it's a resource-intensive intervention?

Overall, research on HACT is making exciting headway. So far, we have learned that adults with severe asthma can benefit from alpine treatment in some way, regardless of phenotype. In addition, many patients experienced lasting improvement for up to twelve months. Be on the lookout as more research is published on this topic.

As always, if you are a patient suffering from asthma, check in with your primary care provider prior to making a trip to altitude to ensure your asthma is well controlled before arrival. While HACT has been shown to decrease asthma symptoms long term, arriving at altitude unprepared and with uncontrolled symptoms could put you at greater risk for high-altitude sickness. As mentioned, cold air can also be a trigger for asthmatics. With that in mind, it may be best to visit the mountains during the summer months. Lastly, always be prepared and carry your rescue inhaler with you, especially when traveling to altitude.

REFERENCES

1. "Asthma | CDC." Centers for Disease Control and Prevention, Centers for Disease Control and Prevention, www.cdc.gov/asthma/default.htm.

2. Fanta, Christopher H. "An Overview of Asthma Management." UpToDate, Helen Hollingsworth, MD, www-uptodate-com.mwu.idm.oclc.org/contents/an-overview-of-asthma-management?search=asthma adult&source=search_result&selectedTitle=1~150&usage_type=default&display_rank=1.

3. Fanta, Christopher H. "Diagnosis of Asthma in Adolescents and Adults." Www, Helen Hollingsworth, MD, www-uptodate-com.mwu.idm.oclc.org /contents/diagnosis-of-asthma-in-adolescents-and-adults?search=asthma definition§ionRank=1&usage_type=default&anchor=H2&source=machineLearning&selectedTitle=1~150&display_rank=1#H3.

4. Fieten, Karin B. et al. "Less Exacerbations and Sustained Asthma Control 12 Months after High Altitude Climate Treatment for Severe Asthma." Allergy, vol. 74, no. 3, 14 Nov. 2018, doi:10.1111/all.13664.

5. Hashimoto, S. et al. "Predictors of Benefit from High-Altitude Climate Therapy in Adults with Severe Asthma." The Netherlands Journal of Medicine, vol. 76, no. 5, July 2018, pp. 218–225.

6. Rijssenbeek-Nouwens, L. H., and E. H. Bel. "High-Altitude Treatment: a Therapeutic Option for Patients with Severe, Refractory Asthma?" Clinical & Experimental Allergy, vol. 41, no. 6, 2011, pp. 775–782., doi:10.1111/j.1365-2222.2011.03733.x.

7. Seys, Sven F et al. "Effects of High Altitude and Cold Air Exposure on Airway Inflammation in Patients with Asthma." Thorax, vol. 68, no. 10, 2013, pp. 906–913., doi:10.1136/thoraxjnl-2013-203280.

8. Vinnikov, Denis et al. "High-Altitude Alpine Therapy and Lung Function in Asthma: Systematic Review and Meta-Analysis." 6.2 Occupational and Environmental Health, 2016, doi:10.1183/13993003.congress-2016.pa4293.

How Altitude Can Permanently Change Your Brain

The brain is a highly demanding organ that requires a constant supply of oxygen, evidenced by how quickly a drowning victim loses consciousness. But it's not just underwater—there are many other environments that expose our brains to the low oxygen levels that cause **hypoxia**, or lack of oxygenated blood flow to the brain. The most common of these is altitudes over 8,000 feet (2,500 meters).

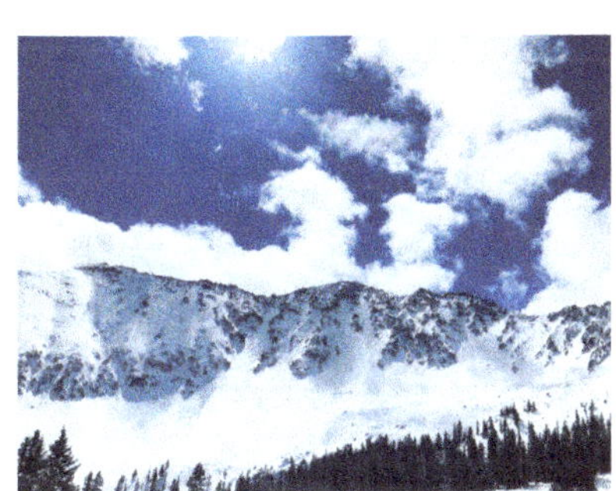

The East Wall of the Continental Divide, above Arapahoe Basin ski area, Colorado.

How does long-term exposure to low oxygen levels in these environments affect our brains? Recent studies have revealed new dangers of exposure to extremely high altitudes—15,000 feet (4,572 meters) and higher—but also suggest our brains feel the impact at less-extreme elevations.

Extremely high-altitude locations are some of the most impressive and breathtaking places in the world, often serving as bucket list checkpoints for travelers and mountaineers everywhere. A 2006 study by Fayed et al. reported a new risk for extremely high-altitude hikers: When MRI scans were performed on the brains of those returning from locations including Mt. Everest, Mt. Aconcagua, Mont Blanc, and Mt. Kilimanjaro, most of the Everest climbers returned with brain changes on their MRI scans, revealing cortical atrophy and enlargement of their Virchow-Robin spaces, processes that are usually associated with aging.[1] The amateur of the group seemed to suffer the most permanent changes with subcortical lesions as well.[1] Where there had been one unaffected hiker in the Everest group, none returned from the Aconcagua expedition without brain changes. Four hikers also showed subcortical lesions.[1] Unfortunately, and even more concerning, most of these changes were still present on MRI scans several years afterward.[1]

A follow-up study in 2015 by Kottke et al. examined mountaineers before and after a 7,126-meter (23,380-foot) ascent and found that none had subcortical lesions.[2] There were increases in cerebral spinal fluid fractions and decreases in white matter fractions in several of the hikers. They also took it a step further and related it to the hypoxic levels and mountain sickness symptoms the individuals suffered and were able to correlate these episodes with more significant brain changes.[2]

Researchers have also found ways to approach altitude that seem to lessen these effects, starting with ascending slowly.[1] Permanent brain changes in extreme-altitude hikers seemed to be worse in the amateurs who had ascended too quickly compared to the professionals who ascended over time.[1] Oxygen supplementation and other methods to prevent acute mountain sickness during the climbs also helped.[1]

Frequent visits to (or residence at) moderately high altitudes can also affect the brain. Abrupt gains in altitude impact memory storage and recall[3] and cause temporary impairment in concentration, a decline in finger-tapping speed, and aphasia.[3] A 2016 study of young, healthy individuals living at altitudes of 3,650 meters (11,976 feet) for a minimum of three years showed significant impairments in attention.[4] Early and late stages of attentional processes were impacted in this study group when compared with a control group.[4] The effects were worsened by larger amounts of perceptual input, or distractions.[4] Attention span data did show impairment in early and late stages, with changes in brain activation on brain scans proposed as possible compensatory mechanisms.[4] This discrepancy lessened the longer the individual lived at altitude, suggesting adaptation was occurring.[4]

For travelers, ascending slowly gives the brain time to acclimatize, decreasing physical and mental symptoms such as confusion, sluggish thinking, or difficulty with concentration and focus.[1] Proper hydration, nutrition, and oxygen supplementation can lessen symptoms as well.

More research is needed to study the effects of permanent brain changes to determine whether there really is a risk of diminished attention span or other cognitive processes from living at high altitude. Although it is important to be aware of these risks, very few residents and adventurers let it hold them back from visiting and living in some of the most incredible places in the world. As long as we approach with an understanding of the dangers, prepare appropriately, and always ascend slowly, not even our brains can hold us back from the adventures to be had in these amazing locations.

REFERENCES

1. Fayed, N., Modrego, P. and Morales, H Evidence of brain damage after high-altitude climbing by means of magnetic resonance imaging. American Journal of Medicine. 2006. 119, 168.e1-168.e6.

2. Kottke, R. Hefti, JP. Rummel, C. Hauf, M. Hefti, U. Merz, TM. Morphological brain changes after climbing to extreme altitudes – a prospective cohort study. PLoS One. 2015; 10(10): e0141097.

3. Hombein, TF. Long term effects of high altitude on brain function. Int J Sports Med. 1992;(13) Supple 1:S43-5.

4. Wang, Y. Ma, H. Fu, S. Guo, S. Yang, X. Luo, P. Han, B Long-term exposure to high altitude affects voluntary spatial attention at early and late processing stages. Scientific Reports. 2014; (4) 4443.

Closer to the Sun: The Dermatological Benefits and Consequences of Living at High Altitude

As many of us know, high-altitude living goes hand in hand with a multitude of outdoor activities, like biking, hiking, and skiing. But with all that outdoor activity comes an insidious risk: radiation from the sun. According to an interview with Kim Guthke, PA-C, a physician assistant working in dermatology in Boulder, Colorado, "living at a higher elevation exposes us to approximately twenty-five percent more ultraviolet radiation when compared to sea level."[1]

Using thick, UV-protective clothing, sunglasses, and sunscreen (and reapplying it) are great ways to protect our skin from the sun. By contrast, in an article from *Outside* magazine called "Is Sunscreen the New Margarine?," Rowan Jacobsen discussed a novel study claiming only the sun can provide the vitamin D we need and that pills just aren't good enough. Vitamin D is required for absorbing calcium, whose levels, if low, can increase one's risk of "cancer, diabetes, obesity, osteoporosis, heart attack, stroke, depression, cognitive impairment, autoimmune conditions, and more."[2] To decrease the risk of these diseases, healthcare workers promote vitamin D supplementation.

But Jacobsen reports that many studies have proven supplementation of vitamin D isn't enough to lower that risk. With normal vitamin D levels, the general health of the patient did not improve. Yet there was also no correlation between high supplemented vitamin D levels and overall health.

Why was this?

Jacobsen claims that vitamin D is actually just a marker for overall health. In other words, raising vitamin D by artificial supplementation does not make one healthier; rather, to raise one's vitamin D level, one must live a healthy lifestyle outside in the sun. Jacobsen states, "What made the people with high vitamin D levels so healthy was not the vitamin itself ... their vitamin D levels were high because they were getting plenty of exposure to the thing that was really responsible for their good health—that big orange ball shining down from above."[2]

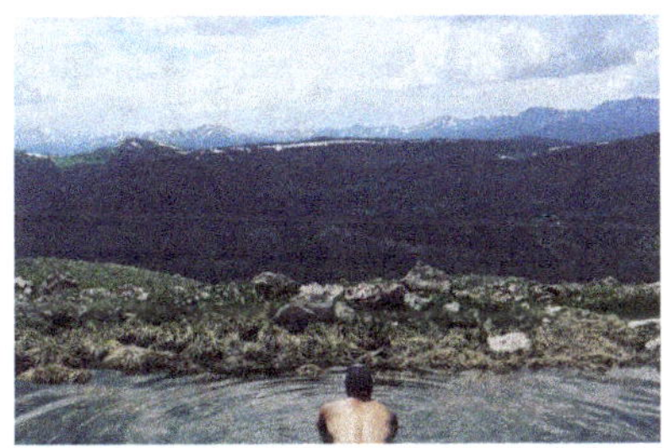

Ice bath on the way up Uneva Peak, off Vail Pass, Colorado.

So, what are the implications of this study? Does this mean we all need to stop using sunscreen in order to absorb the most natural form of vitamin D and subsequently decrease our risk of dangerous diseases? Well, yes and no.

Yes, in that the best way to absorb vitamin D is from the sun, and sunscreen does inhibit that absorption. No, in that a single day of playing at the beach and getting horribly sunburned is not going to improve health. I hypothesize that those living at high altitude don't need as much time to absorb the same amount of beneficial sunlight as those living at sea level, so there is still a need for sunscreen and protective clothing if outside for an extended period.

In his article, Jacobsen admits that increasing sun exposure does increase the rate of skin cancer, but then claims this is "okay" because "skin cancer kills surprisingly few people: less than 3 per 100,000 in the United States each year ... People don't realize this because several different diseases are lumped together under the term 'skin cancer.' The most common by far are basal-cell carcinomas (BCCs) and squamous-cell carcinomas (SCCs), which are almost never fatal."[2]

Dermatological surgeons perform Mohs micrographic surgery, a delicate and precise surgical procedure, to remove these cancers from the face, ears, scalp, fingers, and toes. Although BCCs and SCCs are rarely fatal, they can cause significant damage to one's appearance. Depending on the location and size of the cancer, a "non-fatal" SCC in situ has the potential to cause extensive disfigurement of the face, ears, or eyes. Saying skin cancer is non-fatal creates a false sense of security. This can be especially dangerous at high altitude, where the sun's rays are much stronger than elsewhere in the United States.

Sunshine, at least in moderation, is incredibly beneficial to our health, and the balance between risk and benefit varies between individuals and their skin types. Living in the Colorado mountains gives more opportunities to enjoy the mountain air, along with the sun, and promotes healthier lives in general.

REFERENCES

1. Guthke, Kim. "Sun Protection at Higher Altitudes." Boulder Medical Center, 29 August 2018, www.bouldermedicalcenter.com/sun-protection-at-higher-altitudes.

2. Jacobsen, Rowan. "Is Sunscreen the New Margarine." Outside Online, 6 June 2019 www.outsideonline.com/2380751/sunscreen-sun-exposure-skin-cancer-science?utm_source=pocket&utm_medium=email&utm_campaign=pockethits.

Your Flu Shot Is Even More Important at 9,000 Feet

Winter may be the favorite season for mountain residents until they have to miss out on the fun and work due to influenza. Flu and the common cold are two separate illnesses affecting people more often between November and April that are prevented and treated differently. The common cold is generally a mild and self-limiting viral infection, caused by one of more than two hundred types of viruses from the rhinovirus family.[6] Because of the vast number of viruses responsible for the common cold, there is no vaccine. By contrast, the flu is caused by a smaller family of viruses, influenza A and influenza B.[5] While the flu may also be self-limiting in some cases, it carries a higher risk of severe complications than the common cold and is thus monitored by both the Centers for Disease Control and the World Health Organization.[5]

The flu and common cold share many symptoms, often causing confusion about when to seek medical treatment. Fever is generally higher in influenza infections along with severe headache, body aches, coughing, and even vomiting in children.[2] The only way to know for sure is by testing for flu using a rapid flu swab, which can be done in the clinic. If your flu swab is positive for influenza, antiviral medications, such as oseltamivir, or Tamiflu, can be used to reduce the chances of severe complications.[2]

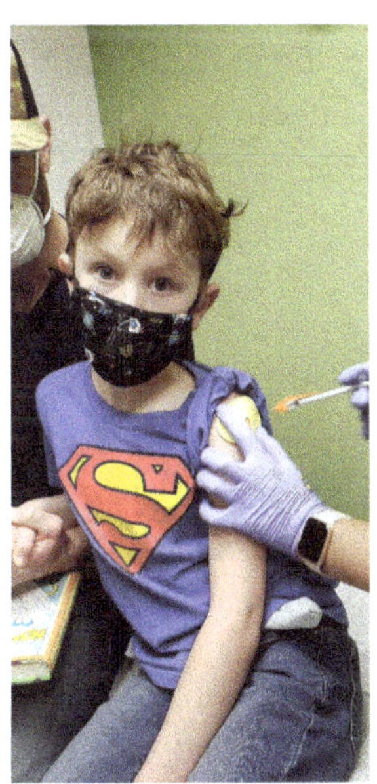

You don't have to be Superman to get your influenza vaccine—it comes as nose drops, too.

Unfortunately, mountain residents are at higher risk of complications from influenza infections. Data gathered from across Mexico during the 2009 H1N1 influenza pandemic showed that rates of hospitalization and death from influenza in patients living above 1,765 meters (5,791 feet) were three times those of patients living below that altitude.[7] Frisco, Colorado, sits at 2,766 meters (9,075 feet) above sea level. While many remember the 2009 flu year as one of the worst in recent history, with 384 pediatric flu deaths in the United States, it should also be noted that every year, over 100 children in the United States die from influenza complications. About 85% of these children are not vaccinated against influenza.[5]

Influenza viruses can lead to death by breaking down epithelia cells found along our airways and even causing macrophages and neutrophils, two types of white blood cells, to malfunction. These attacks on the immune system make the infected victim susceptible to bacterial infections, such as pneumonia.[4] Viral infections like influenza increase the risk of **high-altitude pulmonary edema (HAPE)**.[3] Children aged six months to four years are at an even higher risk of these devastating complications of influenza infection.[4]

Receiving the flu vaccine each year is an easy way to prevent severe flu infections for you and your loved ones. The flu vaccine is available as a nasal mist, adding another layer of protection in the mucous membranes where the virus enters the body. There is no longer any contraindication to flu vaccines for people with allergies to eggs. Pregnant women are especially prone to complications and death from influenza, making vaccination important. The new baby is protected for up to six months from the mother's antibodies after vaccination during pregnancy. All preparations of the flu vaccine are either inactivated influenza virus or recombinant influenza virus (or parts of the DNA from the virus). Neither of these preparations involve live influenza viruses, and they cannot cause an influenza infection.

REFERENCES

1. Centers for Disease Control and Prevention. (2016). Vaccination Who should do it, who should not and who should take precautions. Retrieved from: https://www.cdc.gov/flu/protect/whoshouldvax.htm#flu-shot.

2. Decker, B & Herring, M. (2011). Influenza vs the common cold: Symptoms and treatment. Pharmacy Times, 77(11): 80. Retrieved from: http://go.galegroup.com.libproxy.uccs.edu/ps/i.do?p=AONE&u=colosprings &id=GALE|A305993419&v=2.1&it=r&sid=summon&authCount=1.

3. Hevroni, A., Goldman, A., & Kerem, E. (2015). High altitude: Physiology and pathophysiology in adults and children: A review. Clinical Pulmonary Medicine, 22(3): 105-113. DOI: 10.1097/CPM.0000000000000093.

4. Martin-Loeches, I., Van Someren Greve, F., & Schultz, M. J. (2017). Bacterial pneumonia as an influenza complication. Current Opinion in Infectious Disease, 30(2): 201-207. doi1097/QCO.0000000000000347.

5. Munoz, F. M. (2017). Seasonal influenza in children: Clinical features and diagnosis. In G. B. Mallory & M. S. Edwards (Eds.) UpToDate Database. Retrieved from: https://www.uptodate.com/contents/the-common-cold-in-children-management-and-prevention?source=search_result&search=cold &selectedTitle=2~150.

6. Pappas, D. E. (2017). The common cold in children: Management and Prevention. In M. S. Edwards & M. M. Torchia (Eds.) UpToDate Database. Retrieved from: https://www.uptodate.com/contents/the-common-cold-in-children-management-and-prevention?source=search_result&search=cold &selectedTitle=2~150.

7. Perez-Padilla, R., Garcia-Sancho, C., Fernandez, R., Franco-Marina, F., Lopez-Gatell, H., & Bojorquez, L. (2013). The impact of altitude on hospitalization and hospital mortality from pandemic 2009 influenza a (H1N1) virus pneumonia in Mexico. Salud publica de Mexico, 55(11): 92-95. doi: 1590/S0036-36342013000100013.

"Eructile" Dysfunction at Altitude: Low Barometric Pressures Worsen Discomfort for Those Who Can't Burp

Lucie Rosenthal's journey, captured in her viral Reddit video, sheds light on a lesser-known condition: **retrograde cricopharyngeus dysfunction**, or "no-burp syndrome." What makes her story particularly fascinating is the intersection of this medical condition with the effects of altitude—a factor that significantly influences the body and its functions.

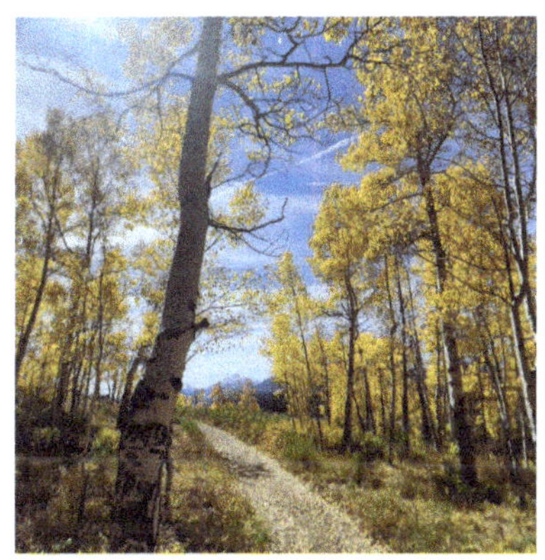

The iconic golden leaves of aspen trees on a Colorado trail in autumn.

In her video, Lucie joyfully discovers her ability to burp after a procedure that injects Botox into the upper esophageal muscle. Her initial excitement turns into an uncontrollable experience that raises questions about the body's mechanisms, especially in relation to altitude. She recounts the bloating and discomfort that accompanies her condition, echoing a broader issue faced by many individuals living at higher elevations, where changes in atmospheric pressure can exacerbate gastrointestinal symptoms.

The relationship between altitude and digestive health is an important consideration. At higher elevations, the reduced atmospheric pressure can lead to gas expansion in the stomach and intestines, intensifying feelings of bloating and discomfort. This is particularly relevant for individuals like Daryl Moody, who struggled with no-burp syndrome while also engaging in activities like skydiving. As he ascended, the altitude caused his stomach to inflate like a bag of chips, amplifying his discomfort and highlighting how altitude can complicate existing health issues.

There is a growing awareness surrounding retrograde cricopharyngeus dysfunction, especially through online communities like the noburp subreddit. These platforms provide vital support for those affected, particularly in regions where altitude impacts digestive health. It's a testament to how individuals can come together to share experiences and coping strategies, transforming personal struggles into a collective understanding of a shared condition.

The financial barriers can be complicated for those living in high-altitude areas. With treatments often deemed "experimental" by insurance companies, individuals may face significant out-of-pocket expenses, particularly in regions where healthcare costs are already high.

Reports of individuals unable to burp date back centuries. The contemporary acknowledgment of retrograde cricopharyngeus dysfunction reflects an evolving understanding of how environmental factors, such as altitude, can play a crucial role in health. As we continue to learn more about this condition, the need for further research into the effects of altitude on digestive health becomes increasingly apparent.

In summary, Lucie Rosenthal's story illustrates the complexities of retrograde cricopharyngeus dysfunction, particularly in relation to altitude. The interplay between physiological responses and environmental factors underscores the importance of patient advocacy and community support in addressing these issues. As we navigate our health, understanding how altitude can influence our bodies highlights the need for a comprehensive approach to medical care that considers all aspects of a patient's environment.

Accessibility at Altitude

How accessible are the places you go?

Volunteers from Ebert Family Clinic in Frisco, Colorado, teamed up with the Northwest Colorado Center for Independence (NWCCI) to join No Barriers, a non-profit program that works to empower people with disabilities and bring communities face to face with what it means to be accessible.

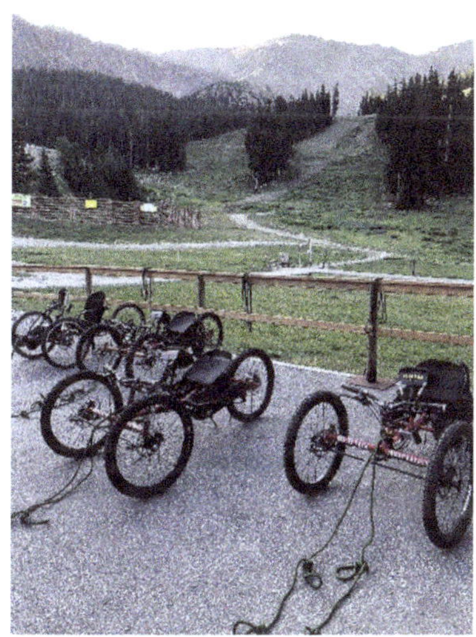

Some of the adaptive equipment provided at the No Barriers hike at Arapahoe Basin. We saw people with all kinds of equipment: hiking poles, one-wheelers, and three-wheelers equipped with every type of pedaling, wheeling, steering, and braking device.

This particular program, called "What's Your Everest," takes place every year at various outdoor venues, connecting people with disabilities with their ropes teams, who assist them in ascending literal mountains. At Arapahoe Basin on the Continental Divide, participants navigated narrow, single-track trails over large rocks, through trees, and up increasingly steep inclines to reach a summit well over 12,000 feet (3,657 meters).

Volunteers and organizations across the state were involved, including STARS (Steamboat Adaptive Recreational Sports), who provided a fleet of adaptive equipment to facilitate the ascent.

I imagine most people associate accessibility with wheelchair access in restaurants, braille menus, audio signaling at crosswalks, and ASL interpreters, but this is just the tip of the iceberg. I promise you have never seen gear like adaptive equipment, and even if you have, you haven't seen all of it.

How do you navigate a wheelchair up a mountain when it's wider than the trail?

How do you operate or steer a wheelchair if you can't grip the wheels or handles?

How do you navigate a trail without sight?

None of this is easy, and even current adaptive equipment has inherent flaws. It's important to recognize that each person's disability is unique and can't always be accommodated by the same piece of equipment produced for the next person.

How do you start thinking about accessibility?

Accessibility is about *cost*. Adaptive equipment is expensive. Custom-making a recumbent bicycle that allows you to pedal without the use of your legs or feet costs thousands of dollars, and people who need this equipment to partake in activities that others without disabilities enjoy should not have to pay more for being disabled.

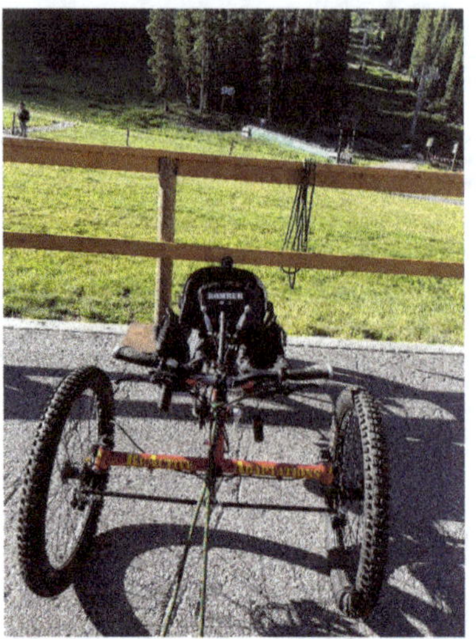

One of a fleet of adaptive cycles that allows riders to steer using pressure against a chest pad while "pedaling" with their hands. You can't brake while using your hands to pedal!

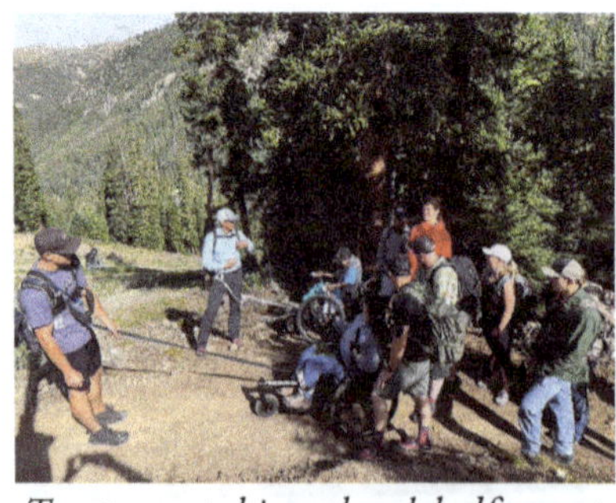

Two teams, taking a break halfway up to Black Mountain Lodge at Arapahoe Basin ski area after navigating some of the narrowest portions of the trail.

Accessibility is about *comfort*. After volunteering at the Colorado Youth Leadership Forum, where young adults with disabilities are empowered and educated about advocating for themselves and living independently, I realized you cannot expect people to stay focused and engaged in your programming if the room is too hot or the provided meal is unfulfilling. If someone without a disability is distracted by the temperature, you can be sure the attention of someone with autism is long gone.

Accessibility is about *time*. However long you think it takes to put on clothes, eat, use the bathroom, or speak a sentence—forget all about it. People with disabilities often need more time. If someone needs more time in the bathroom or walking/wheeling to a destination, adjust your expectations and wait. Your impatience and intolerance will not improve access.

Accessibility is about *language*. Learn sign language. It's just as much a part of our culture as spoken English and Spanish. People with hearing impairments often learn to read lips because they are taught their hearing counterparts can't be bothered to learn a form of communication other than one spoken language. And this isn't just about being deaf. Having a disability sometimes means you have a speech impediment, or that your brain doesn't organize thought and speech the same way others' do.

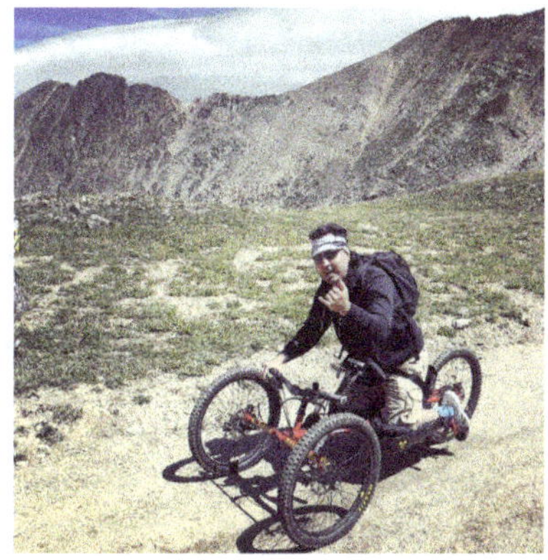

NWCCI Independent Living Coordinator Carlos Santos, hauling down the mountain at Arapahoe Basin ski area on an adaptive cycle after making his ascent to over 12,000 feet (3,600 meters) on foot with hiking poles.

Communicating effectively takes all forms for all disabilities: physical, mental, and emotional.

Accessibility is about *attitude*. Sometimes, people with certain disabilities can be very loud and blunt. Sometimes, they can walk, but with a limp. Sometimes, they speak very slowly. This does not mean they are rude, drunk, can't think for themselves, or can't express their own opinions. Accommodating these situations means being prepared to shift your expectations and perspective.

I've been scolded by people sitting behind me at an opera for whispering translations to my blind companion next to me, before headsets with translations were provided. I've helped my friend into an outdoor trash elevator to get from street level to a downstairs bar. And there was still a step onto the elevator platform. I've witnessed someone being thrown out of a bar for being "too intoxicated," when in reality, he was just paraplegic and walked with a limp. And how is someone in a wheelchair supposed to use a porta-potty at an outdoor music festival?

Is this the best we can do?

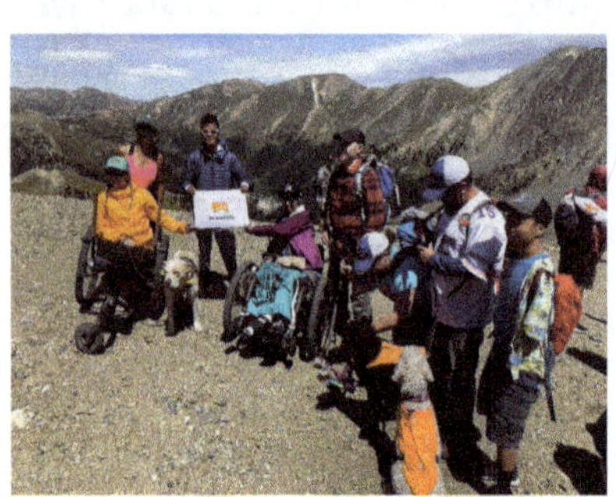

12,500 feet (3,810 meters) after hours of hiking, pushing, pulling, wheeling, and carrying our way to the top of Arapahoe Basin, discovering that "what is inside us is truly stronger than what is in our way."

Our *indoor* establishments are barely held to any minimum standard of accessibility. Why are we doing so poorly, and why does access stop when it comes to the outdoors?

It's important to me that my friends and family with disabilities be able to enjoy the same experiences I do, and I continue to learn more and more about what it means for any event, establishment, activity, or location to be truly accessible and inclusive. I've realized that recommending a place that is "accessible" depends a lot on the disabilities present. Determining whether or not someone in a wheelchair can navigate a trail depends on what kind of wheelchair they're in as well as the grade and width of the trail.

Finally, accessibility is about *problem solving*. It is up to all of us as a community to find solutions that enable our friends and family with disabilities to interact as freely with our environment as those of us without disabilities, both indoors and out. I encourage anyone and everyone to start with a simple visual assessment: take a look around you next time you are on a hike, in a brewery, by the lake, at the farmer's market, or at your favorite coffee shop, and ask yourself if your disabled counterparts would be able to join you. Start there.

PART VII
NEEDS OF NON-HUMANS

Physiology of an Automobile: Cars Need Oxygen, Too!

There are seven establishments up here in Summit County, Colorado, that offer auto maintenance. That means you will be on a waitlist weeks out to schedule any work you need done during peak season. I finally got an appointment at High Country Auto in Frisco after my SUV started shaking when I drove over forty mph (64 km/h). My undercarriage was caked in enough frozen mud and dirt that it was causing the car to rock.

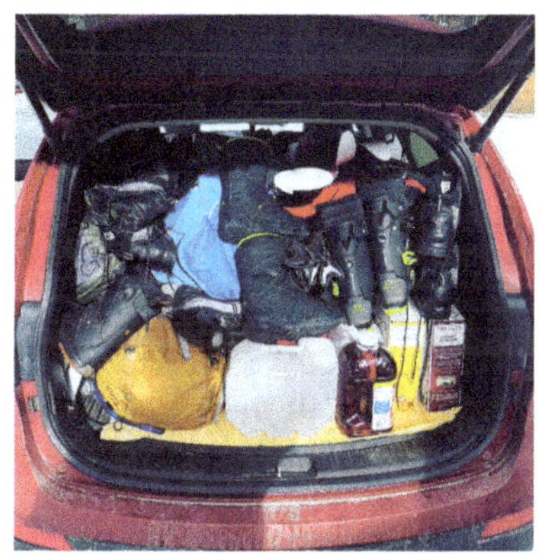

Packed for a winter backcountry excursion!

According to Carrie, who started High Country Auto with her husband, Steve, in 1998, this is a relatively common scenario in the high country. Something else she sees a lot up here is people from sea level putting water in with their washer fluid, which easily freezes on colder days. "The only way to unthaw it is to leave it in the garage overnight," she says.

This prompted more conversation about how cars respond to the extreme altitude, sharp inclines, and lack of oxygen up here.

"A lot of people up here try to run 91 octane, the high-octane gas," Carrie says. "But we don't have enough oxygen up here to burn it. So they gum up their fuel injectors, they gum up their fuel system because they're running too high of octane.

"The other thing people think that they can do is ... 'chip' their car to make it go faster ... they try to bypass parameters on the computer to make it go faster. But it doesn't work up here, because you need to have more oxygen.

"The other problem, too, is that they load their cars down with ten million people and all their [stuff], and then they try to go up the hills. And their car can only go so fast because it can only take in so much oxygen. It can only process so much, plus they're already fully weighted down. And then they hit altitude and their cars are [struggling]." (Insert Carrie's imitation of a car struggling.)

"It's like a big ... 500-pound [227-kilogram] guy going up four stories, and he gets up [to] the first floor and he has a heart attack. Well, why? It's because he's exerting himself at altitude. It's the same thing with cars. If a car has a little bit of a problem up here, and then you load it down with people and you try to get it to go up to 12,000 [3,657 meters], it overworks the car. And a lot of people don't realize that cars have to work harder up here, just like people do."

So, what do you have to do to prepare your car for a trip up to altitude?

"Don't overload it. And don't push your car. Don't try to go faster. When you're going up a hill, be nice to your car. It's like when you're going down a hill, try to go into third gear to let your transmission slow you down. Take your foot off the brakes.

"The problem up here is people try to haul their trailers with Subarus. I've seen fifth wheels being hauled with little tiny cars. It doesn't work up here ... it can't get enough oxygen for the car to process it. The biggest mistake people make up here is they overload everything."

Another little thing you can do to take extra care of your car up here, Carrie says, is let it warm up for two to five minutes when you first start it up in the morning. As the water freezes, all the fluids tend to gel, and it's in your best interest to get these fluids warm again. "When it's twenty below [-29° C], it takes a lot for the car to warm up. Just like us getting out of bed," she laughs.

"This is not the place to push your car. If your car is gonna break down, it's gonna break down up here."

A Survival Guide for Driving the I-70 Corridor

Ah, winter in the Rockies—a magical time of snow-capped peaks, cozy ski lodges, and of course, treacherous driving conditions on Interstate 70. If you're a seasoned local, you know the drill: every time you plan a journey along this notorious stretch of road, you find yourself pondering the eternal question, "When should I brave the chaos of I-70?"

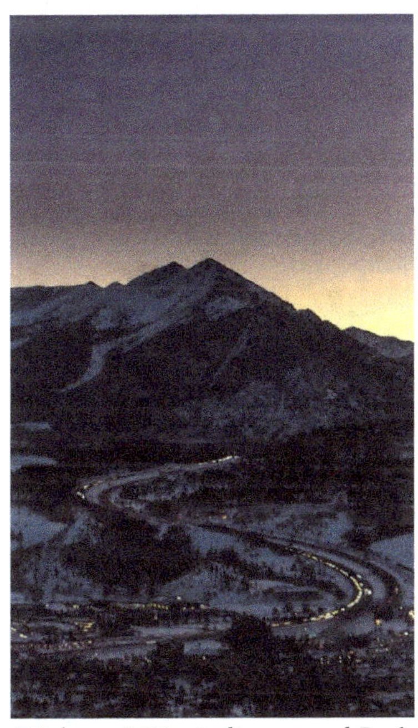

Highway I-70, winding toward Peak One in the Tenmile Range of Colorado at dusk. Photo courtesy of Nate Cordero.

If you value your sanity (and your fender), it's best to avoid I-70 during rush hour, weekends, and holidays. Think of it as trying to navigate through a minefield of impatient tourists and stressed-out locals—a recipe for disaster. And let's not forget about those big snowstorms. While they may turn the landscape into a picturesque winter wonderland, they also transform I-70 into a slippery, white-knuckled nightmare. So, unless you have a burning desire to spend the night in your car, it's probably best to wait until the plows have done their job.

You might be wondering if there's a better time to make the trek to and from the Front Range, the plains east of the central Rockies (like Denver and the airport). Well, the short answer is: not really. But you can prepare a survival kit to help you weather the storm—both literally and figuratively.

First on the list of essentials: water, snacks, a flashlight with charged batteries, blankets that will keep you and your passengers warm in case you're stalled or stuck for twenty-four hours before you reach any kind of indoor accommodations, and a snow and ice scraper for your windows and windshield (even in summer, storms bring snow at high elevations, and most gas stations around the Rocky Mountains will sell these).

Do *not* rely on being able to keep your vehicle running over a long period of time; this is limited by gas (unless your vehicle is a Tesla, in which case it's limited by your electric charge), and falling snow clogging the exhaust pipe of a typical combustion engine can cause carbon monoxide poisoning. You never know when you might find yourself stranded in a snowbank, praying for divine intervention—or at least a passing snowplow. And speaking of emergencies, don't forget the toilet paper for times of desperation. Trust me, when nature calls and there's nowhere to hide, you'll thank me for this invaluable piece of advice. Next up, make sure you have a full tank of gas and extra windshield wiper fluid. Oh, and don't forget the shovel and snow brush.

Let's also talk about vehicle capabilities. If you're lucky enough to own a four-wheel drive (4WD) or all-wheel drive (AWD) vehicle, count your blessings and use it wisely. If not, invest in a set of chains, and more importantly, learn how to put them on *before* you find yourself in a slippery situation. And while we're on the subject, snow tires are worth their weight in gold when it comes to navigating storms on I-70. If you rent a car, make sure it has 4WD or AWD capabilities!

On to some recommendations for staying safe on the road. Take it slow. Don't tailgate. Leave more room than you think behind the person in front of you, because you never know when they might hit the brakes—or the black ice. When traveling downhill, downshift instead of relying on your brakes. And last but not least, don't use cruise control in wet or snowy conditions.

Here are some pro tips from full-time residents of Summit County, Colorado, where there are several ski resorts that see millions of visitors every year:

1. The best days to ski are often just after a blizzard passes, but the *worst* times to commute are during or just after a blizzard passes. If you

see a blizzard coming and want to make the most of your ski trip, push your commute up a day or two and plan to spend the blizzard *at* your accommodations so getting to the fresh snow requires little or no driving. If paying more for an extra day or two of lodging isn't in the budget, then neither is getting into an accident or having to be towed out of a ditch in a blizzard. The chances of you having to pull over or pay for lodging on the way to your destination are too high to make it worth the commute in a blizzard.

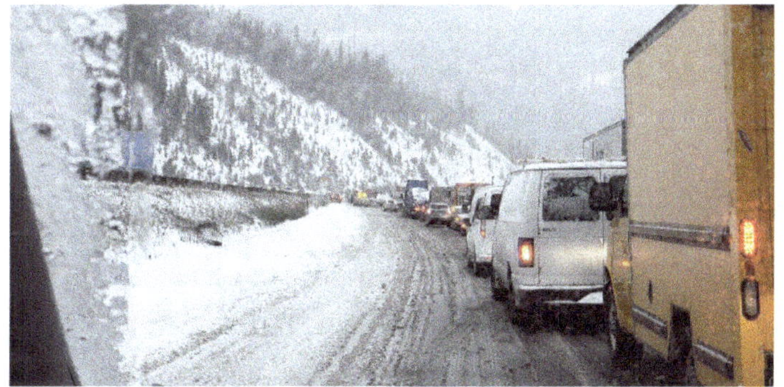
Colorado's treacherous I-70 through the Rocky Mountain corridor.

2. The mountain highway corridors in Colorado are unsurprisingly packed on weekends. Leaving early in the morning or late at night are best for avoiding traffic, but keep in mind there may be more wildlife on the highways when it's darker out, especially in the warmer months. Weekdays are almost always better for avoiding traffic, both on the highway and on the trails.

3. The Colorado Department of Transportation (CDOT) Safety Patrol Program provides some courtesies to motorists that also serve to prevent and relieve traffic congestion in emergencies, including changing flat tires, providing fuel, jump starting vehicles, clearing debris, and more. Their website is one of the most comprehensive resources for your highway travel plans.

4. In the unfortunate event you are caught driving in a storm, snow or otherwise, it is so easy to panic and start worrying you will never see

the end of it. But just like any other weather pattern, it doesn't always maintain the same intensity and will eventually pass. Delays may only be a matter of minutes or hours. So use a reliable app or website to keep tabs on how long it might be before it's safe to proceed. If you insist on driving through a storm, keep your headlights and taillights on. A good rule of thumb is if you cannot see the road markers, you probably should pull over before you end up in a ditch.

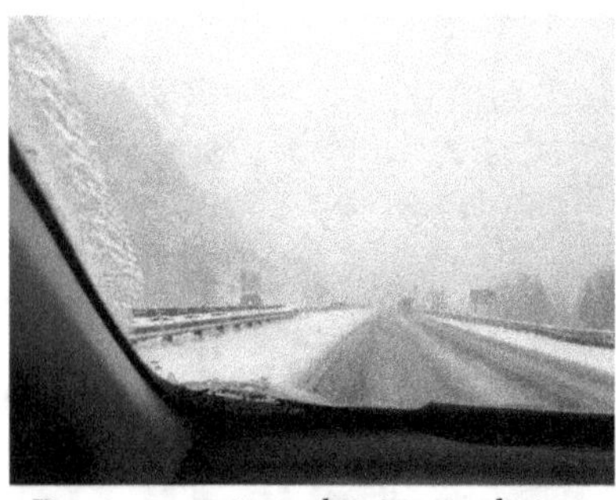

Dangerous winter driving conditions.

5. If you can't see the road markers, it will be tricky to identify a safe place to pull off the road. Instead, observe where other motorists have safely pulled off the road. Large commercial vehicles are more heavily regulated than private vehicles and are expected to be more cautious, and large pullouts are provided to accommodate them along Colorado highways. Look for where those trucks are pulled over while keeping a safe distance.

6. Here's one final pro tip you may never have considered: footwear. You may have gotten into your cozy car wearing slippers or UGGs. But imagine having to get out and change a tire or grab blankets from the trunk in the pouring rain or a foot of snow while wearing those. If the weather's looking unstable, have a pair of shoes or boots you feel comfortable being outside in. (And don't put them in the trunk.)

USEFUL LINKS

- https://www.cotrip.org/home (Weather, road conditions and closures, cameras)
- https://www.instagram.com/i70things
- https://www.codot.gov/programs/dmo/real-time-operations/traffic-incident-management/safetypatrol

Dogs at Altitude

In Colorado, our mountain communities are home to more animals than people. Every spring, we're likely to see everything from foxes to moose in our yards and on our streets. About a month ago, I watched a juvenile—but plenty large—black bear on an evening walk in front of the houses in our neighborhood, peeking into the line of garbage bins that were waiting to be picked up.

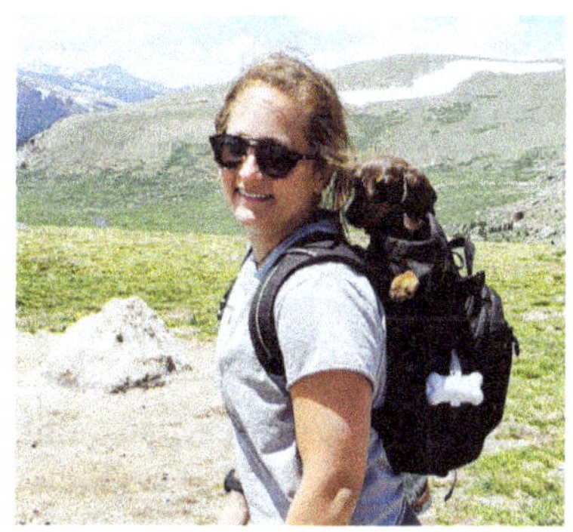

Claire Tinker, with her Dachshund, Baxter, on Mt. Bierstadt.

Dogs are natural companions to many up here as well, with plenty of space to run around, smells to sniff, and communities that seem to welcome their company indoors as well as out. Having seen so many of our dog friends on trails all across the state, we've wondered how they cope with the altitude.

Most recently, we ran into a German Shorthaired Pointer named Moose on an ascent up Mt. Bierstadt, one of Colorado's fourteeners, sitting at 14,060 feet (4,285 meters). He and his human, Nick, moved to Colorado permanently about a year ago, after a two-week visit turned into several months.

Moose is thirteen years old, Nick tells me, "but you have to believe that my dog acts like he's six." Nick and Moose have been enjoying a lot of time outdoors together since moving to Colorado, and Bierstadt was their first fourteener together. They were with some other friends from Louisiana, their home state.

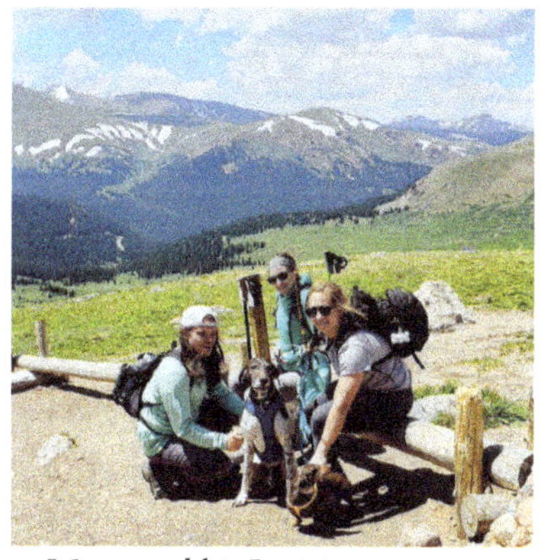

Moose and his Louisiana posse, on their way up Mt. Bierstadt.

For a variety of reasons, many hikers have found themselves carrying their canine counterparts: they get tired, the terrain is difficult for them to negotiate, the ground is too rough on their bare paws, and so on. This is a very legitimate concern. You definitely don't want to have your hands full as you ascend or descend a fourteener.

Dr. Danielle Jehn, who has been a veterinarian with Frisco Animal Hospital for years after studying and practicing in Nebraska, recommends waiting to take your puppy on the longer, more strenuous hikes.

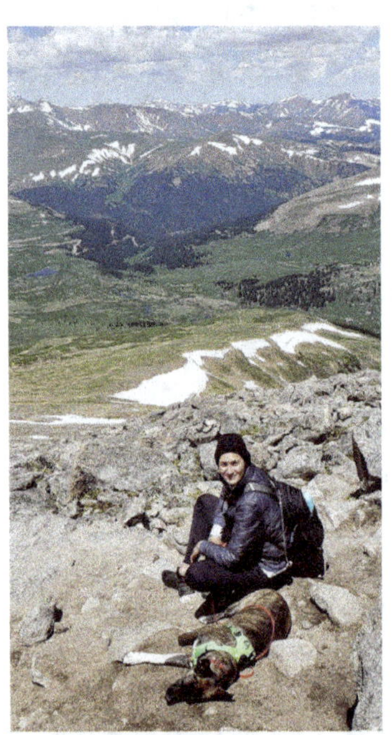

Ike, about eight months old, seriously reconsidering his choices on his way up Mt. Bierstadt.

"Unfortunately, we do not get a chance to discuss this with many owners unless there are new puppy owners. Usually, we just see the aftermath from a hike and help guide them for future incidents. I would love to be able to tell all new puppy owners that activity needs to be limited up until six to eight months of age while they are experiencing enormous amounts of bone growth. This means no major hikes on uneven surfaces and no ten-mile [16-kilometer] runs while the owner mountain bikes. We just want the pups to grow normally without complications for them or the owners."

As you might have speculated, animals are also prone to certain risks at high altitudes, although "in general, healthy animals do not function any differently at high altitude," says Dr. Jehn. "Animals and pets with known blood pressure, cardiac, or respiratory disease can decompensate at higher altitudes, and we do see this in practice. Just as human hearts have a difficult time at altitude, so do cats, dogs, and livestock!"

So, how do you know if your furry buddy is struggling with acclimation?

"Most often, an owner will call and have a presenting complaint of their pet experiencing exercise intolerance while on a hike, or constant panting, lethargy, or anorexia since the pet has been up in Summit County. If a dog presents in any type of respiratory distress, we place them on supplemental oxygen, check their heart and lung sounds, heart rate, respiratory rate, blood pressure, and ability to oxygenate. We do this by utilizing a tool in the clinic that measures the percentage of oxygen carried in the blood." Sound familiar? "We always want to see a dog at over 92%. If the dog or cat cannot maintain that or better without being provided oxygen, we need to see other diagnostics for reasons why.

"Common canine ailments we see that are drastically exacerbated by altitude are: cardiac disease (heart murmur, pulmonary hypertension, congestive heart failure), general hypertension, lung disease (asthma, allergic bronchitis), or vascular volume abnormalities (anemia, for example)."

The most common injuries Dr. Jehn sees, she tells me, are "lacerations and abrasions from the rough terrain. We also see exacerbated lameness after hikes that are too long for our canine friends that are not otherwise used to it (for example, fourteeners)."

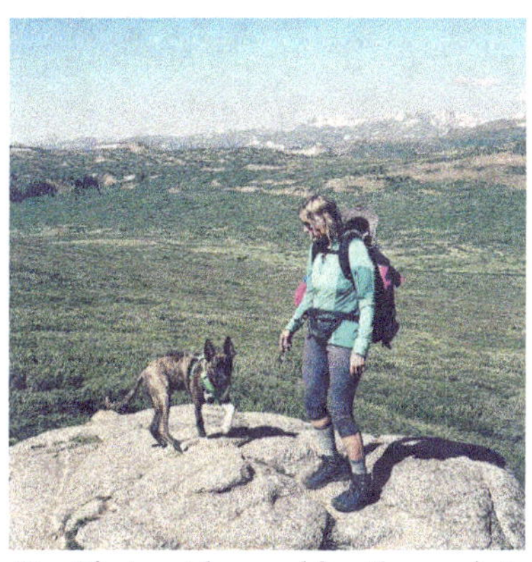

Dr. Chris, with granddog Ike, on their way up Mt. Bierstadt.

Nick and Moose currently live in Boulder, at 5,328 feet (1,624 meters), but they moved there from a house in Bailey, at about 7,740 feet (2,359 meters). I ask Nick if Moose has ever had trouble with the altitude since they moved to Colorado.

"Not at all. Not even when we first got here. He was ready to rock and roll. The only thing he didn't like was the snow at first. Once he realized there were rabbits and stuff that went in the snow, he was about it."

Being from Louisiana, one of Moose's greatest challenges is the relative scarcity of water. Colorado doesn't have as many lakes and ponds that Moose can cool off in and drink from, so Nick says he's sure to carry water for him.

Another factor that affects both Moose and humans is exposure. "If there's no shade or wind, it's a lot harder on him," Nick notes. "We also relate over the challenge of descending a mountain, when the resistance of gravity is especially stressful on your knees and hips."

Nick works for Sacred Genetics, a company that cultivates feminized hemp seeds. They partner with another company, Verdant Formulas, that specializes in CBD products, utilizing the relaxing, remedial properties of the oil from cannabis. Among other applications, balms and oils infused with CBD have grown in popularity as a naturopathic treatment for muscle soreness and inflammation. Increasingly, similar products are being marketed for the same afflictions in dogs. Nick tells me they help with his own post-adventure soreness.

My main takeaway from all this insightful doggo dialogue is that whether we're talking about people or dogs, the same precautions apply for avoiding a serious situation outdoors. Remember, if anyone in your party is having trouble on your hike, it is not advisable to continue; you are only as strong as the weakest member of your team, whether that's a dog or a person.

A last bit of advice from Dr. Jehn:

"I would also love to be able to tell all tourists to take it easy on their canine counterparts while visiting us in Summit County as well. Altitude sickness is real for humans and dogs alike. Accomplishing a crazy hike with your dog should not be the first priority within the first few days at elevation. Dehydration and prior health conditions are real when experiencing altitude. If you know your dog has a history of a heart or lung issue, especially let them take it easy. We want you to enjoy Summit County for everything it has to offer ... without the emergency visit!"

Dogs and the High-Country Winter

Dr. Margot Daly, DVM, CCRP, CVA, of the Frisco Animal Hospital in Frisco, Colorado, graduated from the University of California, Davis, in 2013, and has worked in general practice, emergency practice, and most recently in specialty practice as a full-time rehabilitation and sports medicine veterinarian. Prior to veterinary school, she studied sociology at UC Berkeley and had a career as a professional equestrian, which led to an interest in orthopedics, biomechanics, and physical rehabilitation. Following graduation, she received the Certified Canine Rehabilitation Practitioner designation from the University of Tennessee, Knoxville, and the Certified Veterinary Acupuncturist designation from the Chi Institute in Reddick, Florida. She has been with the Frisco Animal Hospital for a year and a half, and when she is not working, she can be found riding a horse or one of her many bicycles, fostering dogs and kittens, reading books, skiing, or traveling somewhere new.

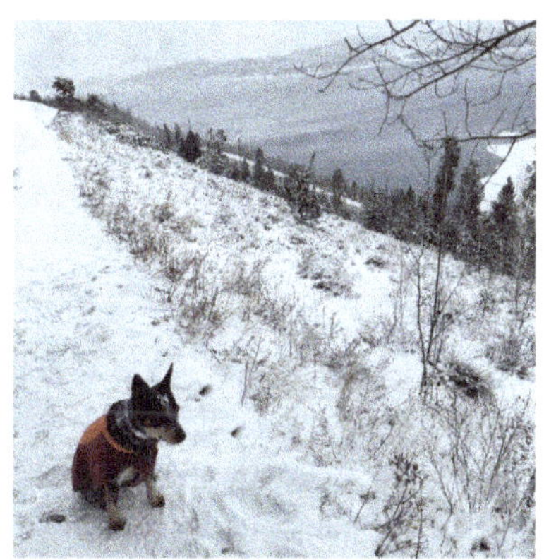

Blue Heeler Isa is ready for anything on a Colorado trail in winter.

We interviewed Dr. Daly and asked for her advice on canine high-country health, winter dog gear, common winter injuries, and winter activities to participate in with your dog.

One of the most common things to be aware of, Dr. Daly says, is canine "weekend warrior syndrome." Dog owners must be sure their dogs are fit enough to participate in physically intense weekend activities. Many dogs only go out in their yards or take a few short walks during the week and then go on big hikes, backcountry ski trips, or long mountain-bike rides on the weekends. Unfortunately, during this high-intensity activity, the dog's adrenaline is high, and while the dog won't show signs of fatigue, the next day the dog will feel awful and be extremely sore. It's comparable to a human doing CrossFit only once a week—imagine how he or she would feel the next day. To avoid this phenomenon, ensure your dog is fit enough by practicing thirty to sixty minutes of moderate exercise at least three times a week, which can include thirty minutes of jogging or sixty minutes of active walking. If your dog is doing less than that during the week, it's important to be thoughtful of what you're asking of your dog or what you are giving it the opportunity to do over the weekend. Unfortunately, a fun weekend can become overly taxing on your dog very quickly.

Signs your dog may have done too much over the weekend include not wanting to go up or down stairs, refusing to jump in and out of the car, and not wanting to get up or down from the couch. Your dog may not necessarily be limping; general full-body fatigue, aches, and soreness are more likely. If your dog isn't eating and drinking normally, that is a reason to call your vet.

WINTER CLOTHING & GEAR

BOOTIES

Dog clothing can be helpful, as dogs get cold just like humans do during outdoor winter activities. Booties can be advantageous during both summer and winter activities. The best policy is to pay attention to your dog's behavior to determine how necessary booties are. Some dogs make it clear they are uncomfortable in the snow and slush by holding their paws high in an alternating fashion, sitting down, or refusing to walk. Some dogs are more sensitive than others, and some have a higher tolerance for cold than others.

The key to booties is acclimating your dog over a week or so before taking the booties out on an adventure. The best way to do this is to put the new booties on your dog in your house, then let your dog have a treat or play with its favorite toy. This will help reinforce the booties and make them a fun experience for your dog. It may take several days before the dog will tolerate the booties and walk around comfortably in them. Essentially, don't wait until the morning of the big hike to put the booties on your dog for the first time.

Another strategy is to start with lightweight booties made of felt with one Velcro strap. These are a cheap, lightweight option and are the same booties sled dogs use on the Iditarod. It's best to buy a few sets of these to start, as some will inevitably get lost. If you find your dog requires something more substantial, Dr. Daly recommends Ruffwear boots, which have heavy rubber soles. Be aware these booties may cause difficulty for dogs with mobility issues, impairing their ability to walk safely. Custom booties are also an option and are recommended for dogs with atypically shaped feet, such as greyhounds. A company called Thera-Paw will coordinate with your vet to get measurements of your dog's feet and make custom booties.

If your dog is totally intolerant of booties—but could benefit from them—you can try musher wax. It provides a slightly waterproof barrier between your dog's paws and the road. It also helps prevent ice balls in dogs with a lot of feathering on their paws or between their toes. Put the wax on right before you take your dog outside and wipe the dog's paws as soon as you get home. This protects dogs from salt, sand, and ice chemicals on the road.

JACKETS

Dr. Daly confirms there are dogs who may benefit from jackets, especially when participating in winter hiking or backcountry skiing. If you see your dog shivering, hunching its back, or crouching its neck and shoulders, your dog is likely cold and would benefit from a jacket. It's imperative to choose a jacket with a full chest and short sleeves over one that just has a strap across the chest. This ensures that the snow will slide off the chest and not become trapped against the dog's skin. It's hard for a dog to overheat in the winter, so it's a good idea to provide layering for your dog. Most importantly, don't choose a cotton fabric, but a fabric that will wick and dry quickly, such as fleece, soft shell, or technical fabric. If your dog's jacket gets wet, be sure to take it off, because a wet jacket is no longer providing warmth and will end up making your dog colder.

GOGGLES

There are many canine patients with eye problems related to increased UV light exposure at high altitude. In particular, pannus, an eye condition exacerbated by UV light, is common in dogs living at high altitude. This immune-mediated condition affects the cornea and causes pink or gray granular tissue to grow from the lateral cornea toward the medial cornea. It is a type of chronic superficial keratitis that certain breeds, specifically German Shepherds, are more prone to. For this reason, goggles are recommended for dogs living at high altitude, especially if the dog is a high-risk breed or if it's already been diagnosed with pannus. Weekend warriors are at a much lower risk of developing pannus, so goggles are not as strongly recommended.

As with booties, dogs must be acclimated to goggles with treats or playtime. Trying out goggles for the first time on the mountain is not recommended. Aim for about a week of acclimation around the house and neighborhood so your dog tolerates the equipment well. Dr. Daly recommends Rex Specs, which do not require a vet to supply measurements, and says she is always happy to help owners measure their dogs.

SUNSCREEN

Surprisingly, canine sunburn is rare, even at high altitude. If it does occur, the burn is normally anywhere the dog has thin to no hair, or pink to white skin. Most commonly it occurs on the nose and belly, especially if the dog prefers to lounge on its back in the sun. Mineral-based sunscreens with an active ingredient of titanium dioxide, such as California Baby, are recommended. After putting sunscreen (or any ointment) on a dog's nose, it's a good idea to immediately give the animal a treat or chew toy so it doesn't lick the ointment right off.

PREVENTION AT HIGH ALTITUDE

The best thing you can do to keep your pet healthy and happy at altitude is ensure adequate hydration. Bring as much water for your dog as you do for yourself. Dr. Daly does not recommend supplemental electrolytes. She also urges owners not to depend on mountain streams, rivers, lakes, snow, or puddles to provide adequate hydration for active high-country dogs, as these natural water sources can contain giardia and leptospirosis. Giardia can cause gastrointestinal symptoms, while leptospirosis can cause liver and kidney failure and has the potential to be transmitted to humans.

Signs your dog may be dehydrated include lethargy, decreased appetite, odd behavior, headshaking, crying out, or barking. Dogs normally tend to drink more water while at altitude, and this behavior is only concerning if the dog has blood in its urine, appears to be in pain while urinating, or is having accidents in the house when it was previously housetrained.

Lastly, if you go camping with your dog, it is imperative you bring your dog's daily medications with you and not skip a day simply because you are camping. Chronic medications can't be skipped for even one dose.

COMMON HIGH-ALTITUDE DIAGNOSES

Dr. Daly sees many recreational injuries and ACL tears between February and April. During this time of year, the snow has a crusty top layer with soft snow underneath. This leads to dogs punching through the top layer and injuring themselves when the soft snow underneath gives way. This postholing causes many ligament strains and tears this time of year. In the beginning of winter, when conditions are predominantly slippery and icy, Dr. Daly sees wrist and toe strains and sprains from dogs trying to grip with their feet.

Another common type of injury is lacerations from backcountry skis. Many people enjoy taking their canine companions backcountry skiing but fail to train the dogs to stay behind them while cruising down the slope. As a result, dogs suffer lacerations from making contact with the skis while running in front of or beside their owners. This can lead to lacerations on the lower legs and around the tendons. Dogs should also be trained to stay behind their owners while mountain biking. Many dogs end up with injuries from running in front of or beside their owners' bikes.

Acute mountain sickness (AMS), high-altitude pulmonary edema (HAPE), re-entry HAPE, or high-altitude cerebral edema (HACE) are exceedingly rare in dogs. The only dogs predisposed to breathing problems are those coming from sea level with underlying cardiac or pulmonic pathologies, such as heart failure or a pulmonary contusion. When coming from sea level with an older dog or one with an underlying comorbidity, Dr. Daly recommends stopping in Denver for two or three nights to let the dog acclimate to the altitude and resultant lower oxygen concentration. Dogs can be prescribed home oxygen concentrators, but these should only be used under the supervision of a veterinarian, as they require a specific home kennel or tubing sewn onto the dog. If your pet falls into a high-risk category, Dr. Daly considers "head pressing"—described as a dog leaning headfirst into a wall, furniture, or other upright object as though it is using the object to hold its head up—as an alarm sign requiring an emergency call to a local vet. Other concerning signs include severe lethargy, vomiting or diarrhea that does not resolve within twenty-four hours, and respiratory distress of any kind.

STRENGTHENING & EXERCISE

Most dogs will benefit from some degree of core and hind limb strengthening, as well as exercises to improve proprioception, or body awareness. The stronger and more coordinated the dog is, the lower its risk of injury, even with high-impact activities. Additionally, dogs can benefit from a personalized exercise program based on unique traits such as a long back, short legs, or preexisting injuries. Dr. Daly's background in sports medicine allows her to assess any dog and provide a program to prevent future—and more importantly, repeat—injuries. If an owner is hoping that his or her companion can return to hiking fourteeners after a ligament tear, then a home exercise program is imperative. Plans generally require about twenty minutes of treatment, three times a week, and incorporate everyday activities such as walking on stairs and working the dog on alternative surfaces. This ensures dog owners won't unnecessarily invest in additional equipment.

BEST WINTER DOG SPORTS CLUBS

Dr. Daly has found that many active dogs enjoy a variety of mushing sports in the winter. These include everything from single- or double-dog skijoring, bikejoring, and canicross (a version of cross-country running with your dog), all the way to dogsledding with two or more dogs. The Colorado Mountain Mushers is a great place to start for anyone interested in exploring these activities. Counting retired professional veterans and amateur mushers among its members, it is a friendly, welcoming, all-inclusive group with abundant resources and advice. The club usually runs about four events each year and can help you learn new ways to connect with your canine companion—huskies not required!

**PART VIII
ALTITUDE EXPERTS**

Doc Talk: The Art of Saving Vacations

In 1986, **Dr. David Gray** was asked to join a team of rafters on an exploration of the Yangtze River in China. Their goal was simple: to reach the undiscovered source of the river and raft all the way down. "Simple" is quite the understatement, though. The Yangtze River is the third-longest river in the world, and the source of the river is approximately 19,000 feet (5,791 meters) above sea level.

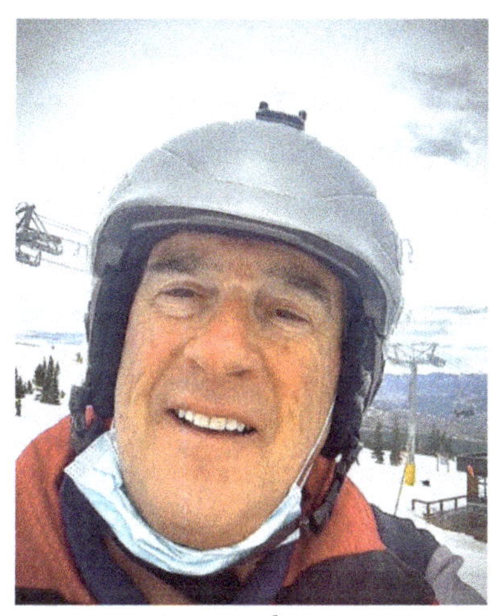
Dr. David Gray.

Dr. Gray, a young physician at the time, agreed to join the mission after being told by the mission frontman, Ken Warren, "We want you there for trauma." Dr. Gray had an inkling the high elevation could present some interesting challenges. He consulted with two pulmonologists, but at the time, understanding of treatment at high altitude was limited, and he got little advice. With eagerness and reassurance that he would "have the final say on all things medical," he began the mission.

The team was an eclectic group of men. With four Chinese Olympic athletes and a cameraman from National Geographic, the crew set forth to uncharted territory. They took a bus up the first 14,000 feet (4,300 meters) and quickly learned about the effects of altitude. "Everyone was sick," Dr. Gray recalls. "I'm treating headaches with narcotics, treating vomiting with phenadrine, and guess what I had for pulmonary edema? Lasix!" Despite the chaos, everybody improved, and the crew trudged forward.

During their slow ascent, they reached a point where the snow was nearly six feet (1.8 meters) deep and vehicles were no longer an option. The rest of the mission would be on foot. With yaks carrying their gear, the crew moved up the glacier to what they presumed was the source of the river. The photographer from National Geographic, David Schippe, had not been doing well. As the mission progressed, Dr. Gray could hear crackles in the base of his lungs through a stethoscope and sent him down to receive medical attention. This was a case of high-altitude pulmonary edema (HAPE), but he was diagnosed with pneumonia.

The rest of the crew reached the presumed source, Tiger Leaping Gorge, which turned out to be one of the many Yangtze tributaries. On their descent down on "duckies" (blow-up rafts), they stopped at base camp and found David Schippe, the photographer who was supposed to have headed back to receive medical care. Their next checkpoint was at 11,000 feet (3,300 meters), 600 miles (965 kilometers) away, and they had no choice but to continue down with Schippe alongside.

Unfortunately, this would be David Schippe's last journey. "On the second day, Schippe started coughing. He got very sick and was put on IV. I said, 'We need the helicopter,' but there was no helicopter. That was all a lie. [Ken] had a shortwave radio, but he used the money for the emergency helicopter to pay his mortgage." Dr. Gray, feeling the weight of this terrible deception, knew this would be the end of Schippe's life. "We buried him on the river," he says.

Dr. Gray distinctly remembers Ken Warren, the expedition leader, announcing their crew member's death. "He said, 'Dave's dead. Suck it up, or you could be next.'"

That was confirmation to Dr. Gray that this mission was being run with no regard for crew safety. When they got to their checkpoint, Dr. Gray said *adios*.

And so went Dr. Gray's introduction to altitude medicine.

Fast forward to today, in a local brewery. Dr. Gray, equipped with the wisdom of twenty years of practice in Summit County, Colorado, and twenty-five years of emergency medicine in Corpus Christi, Texas, shares some essential knowledge for working in the hypoxic conditions of high altitude. An advocate for accessible and affordable healthcare, much of his practice involves bringing medical services straight to his patients.

Has anything changed about what you put in your medical bag since you first started doing mobile healthcare?

No. I had a select group of medications I use that cover almost everything. I get an antibiotic prescription so I can hand them their Z-Pak (my go-to medication). I carry Ventil, Decadron, Nubain (a synthetic narcotic that has some narcotic antagonist effects, so you have to be careful if you put someone using opioids on it, because it'll put them in immediate withdrawal), Benadryl, and epinephrine.

First case of HAPE in Summit County?

He was from Scotland, or somewhere in the British Isles. I sent him to the hospital. He got in the ambulance, spent two days in the ICU in Denver, and $30,000 later, they sent him back up!

(**Dr. Christine Ebert-Santos** notes that even physicians in Denver aren't always familiar with high-altitude care and can order extensive testing for symptoms that are classic presentations of HAPE.)

I got a guy from Austin. He was in his late forties. He had pulmonary edema, and his O$_2$ [saturations] were maybe in the 70s. I said, "You need to go to the hospital. Get out of the altitude and go to Denver." He said, "I don't want to leave my family. Do I have to leave?"

I told him, "I'm going to work with you, but you have got to do everything I say. I'll be back in the morning to give you another dose of Decadron, and you don't get to sue me if this doesn't end well."

I see him the next day, give him another shot of Decadron. He was one of the first people I allowed to stay at altitude. I wouldn't leave anybody with that treatment if I couldn't get him up to the high 70s.

Dr. Gray typically puts these patients on oxygen full time at approximately five liters, monitors them closely, and finds patients' oxygen saturations will typically go up into the 90s. "I got confident with what I was doing," he says.

It's essential to recheck vitals in these patients and pay attention to symptoms, Dr. Gray says. Too often, patients present with acceptable oxygen saturations, around 93%, and end up coming back hypoxic. "The oxygen can present in the normal range initially because patients are hyperventilating," he says. "The respiratory muscles cannot maintain that work of breathing, and later their oxygenation will drop."

Dr. Gray and his family also had their own experience with re-entry HAPE:

We were back in Texas for a few weeks. I took them to the [alpine slide] back in Breckenridge, and [my son] Dillon, who always got headaches, comes up to the car and throws up a bunch of red vomit. I told his sister, 'Please tell me he drank a red soda before this.' (He had.) Then we go home and he's just feeling bad. I just figured, it's his headache, or it's a viral bug. Then, luckily, I put him in bed with me. At about ten p.m. that night, he was coughing so much it was keeping me up. I put a stethoscope on him, and it was like a washing machine. His oxygen was 38!

I put him on five liters of oxygen, and he quit coughing. The cough reflex was there because the lungs were trying to do anything to get more oxygen.

It's not that the pulmonary edema was getting better quickly, necessarily. It took about three days for him to get better.

"It ain't about water, it's diet."

What I believe happens when you come two miles in the sky as abruptly as people do: Most Americans are dehydrated anyway. When they get here, the body goes into defense mode. It shunts blood and oxygen into your heart and kidneys, and consequently ... away from your stomach. Then, [visitors] eat restaurant-portion meals and greasy steaks on vacation. That's why vomiting is sometimes the primary symptom.

What I tell people is if you stop in a restaurant on your way up here, choose high-carb, low-fat, low-protein meals. Carbs are easy to transport through the system. Choose smartly, eat half of what they put on your plate, and take the rest home. The last meal should be at five p.m.

Also, alcohol is a mild diuretic at best. The real issue is that it's a respiratory depressant. If you need to drink on this trip, drink in the morning!

Who gets acute mountain sickness?

Young, fit males. They come up here with a resting pulse of fifty-two beats per minute. A well-exercised person can't get their heart rate up to counteract hypoxia. Then they ignore their symptoms because that's what athletes do. As for athletes, I've given up on that. They go one hundred percent, and they are not going to hold back.

Dr. Gray also emphasized seasonal factors:

We see a marked difference in acute mountain sickness in winter and summer. You are by necessity in a hypermetabolic state in the cold. Your body is working hard using oxygen to stay warm. Plus, people are overusing muscles they haven't used all year. In the summer, they come up in cars and meander up. In the winter, they fly and ascend within hours.

[Ages ago], you didn't see any altitude sickness because they came on donkeys—very slowly!

And if you're not sick by day two, you probably won't be.

By the age of fifty ...

Everyone who lives here should sleep on oxygen. If you haven't been here for generations, you need to be on nighttime supplemental oxygen. The only exception to this is in COPD [chronic obstructive pulmonary disease] patients, due to oxygen deprivation driving respiration and CO_2 retention.

I tell full-time residents, 'You need an oxygen concentrator.' It's a nighttime problem. During the day, you're ventilating. At night, you go into a somnolent state, and your breathing goes down.

Muscles are healthier when you use them. That goes for the heart, too. [Summit County residents] are hyperdynamic, cardiac-wise. If you supplement with oxygen at night, you keep the process of pulmonary hypertension from developing.

Advice to the Traveler

Diamox: it changes your acid-base chemistry, acidifying your serum, which essentially turns you into your own ventilator. Some people are aware of their increased respiratory depth, and it may bother them. 125 mg twice a day, beginning two days before travel. Any dose greater than that will just increase side effects.

The water issue: you can't make up for chronic dehydration during the day. The biggest loss of fluid from the human body is insensible loss, moisturizing the air you breathe. Altitude also produces diuresis, as well as a lot of intestinal gas. The poor bacteria in your [gastrointestinal tract] are also hypoxic.

Dr. Gray opened his own practice in Breckenridge, Colorado, caring primarily for travelers. With the motto "We Save Vacations," he expresses a true passion for his practice and the high-altitude population he serves. He developed his practice by networking closely with local ski industry workers—from "lifties" to ski shop employees—and providing fee-for-service immediate care to his patients.

Athletes vs. Amateurs: More Observations of an Altitude Expert

Ski America is a company that has organized accommodations and itineraries for international athletes and vacationers at ski areas around Colorado since 1988. The Omori family, Ski America's founders, lead their clients on tours of Colorado's most renowned mountains, including Aspen (8,040 feet, or 2,450 meters), Beaver Creek (8,100 feet, or 2,469 meters), Vail (8,120 feet, or 2,475 meters), Keystone (9,280 feet, or 2,828 meters), Breckenridge (9,600 feet, or 2,926 meters), Copper (9,712 feet, or 2,960 meters), and Arapahoe Basin (10,780 feet, or 3,286 meters).

Jimi Omori started Ski America as a tour operator for Japanese skiers and snowboarders, and **Ryoko Omori** joined in 2005. Now more than a tour operator, Ski America assists anyone from first-time skiers as young as three to professional racers. With over thirty years of experience guiding amateur skiers and international athletes alike, the Omoris have made fascinating observations of how people adjust to the high-altitude environment of the Rocky Mountains. Ryoko shared some of their valuable insight and experience with me over a cup of tea.

How long do your clients typically stay at altitude?

We have two different kinds of customers. In November until early December, we have a lot of Japanese racers from Japan. They are high school kids, college students. They stay two to four weeks here, in Frisco or Copper Mountain. Then from December to April, we have clients from Japan who stay in Vail or Aspen. Most of them are senior skiers, over sixty years old. They stay about a week in Vail or Aspen. Six nights is very average.

How often do you get repeat customers?

Quite a lot. Not all of them come back every year, but more than once. I would say 70%.

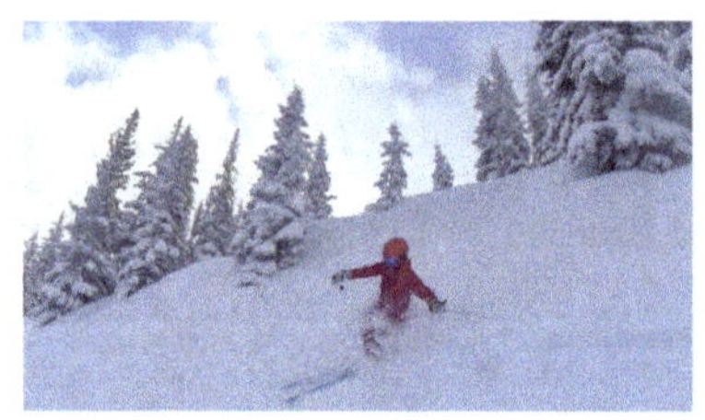

A young skier shreds her way down a snowy back bowl at Vail ski area on a powder day.

Do you see new customers every year?

Yes.

How do you advertise in Japan?

Word of mouth.

How do you prepare your customers for the altitude?

When I set up the reservation for them, I send them the lodging confirmation and shuttle confirmation, and how to get to the Colorado Mountain Express counter at Denver International Airport. With that information, I also send how to get ready for this altitude by e-mail to every customer: Don't stay up all night before coming over here, don't overwork before coming here. Most importantly, don't catch a cold before coming over here. That's the most important thing. And keep yourself hydrated on the flight and on the shuttle. You can always stop at a restroom on the way from the airport to get here. Do not drink a lot [of alcohol] on the flight, and especially on the first night staying here. I encourage them to drink two liters of water a day.

They are so excited to be here, so they tend to forget about the altitude because there are all the trees. It's not above the tree line here. In Japan, [this elevation] is way over the tree line. So I always remind them, "You are going to be almost [at the elevation of] Mt. Fuji. So, move slowly the first and second day of staying here."

What about conditioning and physical exercise to prepare? Are they athletic?

They're pretty much athletic. They're avid skiers. They ski in Japan regularly. So I do not give them any athletic advice in Japan.

Do they come straight from Denver up to elevation, or do they stay in Denver a certain amount of time?

No. The flight arrives at 12:30 or 1 p.m., so it's very convenient for them to get on the shuttle in the afternoon, and they will be here before 5 or 6.

Do they ski the next day?

Most of them, yes.

What about oxygen or medication? Do you ever tell them to bring ibuprofen or anti-nausea medication?

No. But if anything happens here, I recommend taking [something] for a headache, like Advil.

What is the earliest sign that something might be wrong or that they need medical attention?

Headache. Or sometimes nausea. We had 150 racers last November, and out of 150, I took 5 kids to the clinic for altitude sickness symptoms.

Is it at the beginning of their stay?

Very beginning. [Typically] the second day of skiing. They are okay on the first day. They do not notice anything on the first morning, so they feel, "It's okay, let's go skiing!" and spend the day on the mountain, and they have jet lag, and they can't sleep well on the second night. And on the second morning, most of them notice the symptoms. Those are the Copper clients. And I have 350 guests from Japan staying in Vail and Aspen. Last year, I didn't see anyone get sick. So it's only in Summit County, because it's much higher.

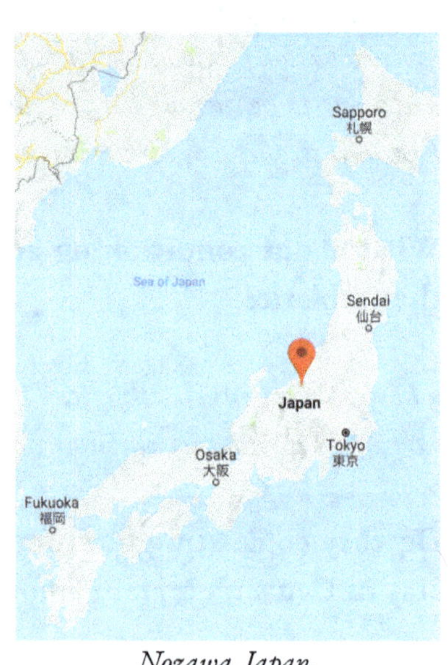

Nozawa, Japan.

Do you think there are any other correlating factors, like their age or where they're from?

Age. The racers are from middle school to college, so they're young. Their hormone level is not stable. And they are staying with their other teammates, apart from their parents, so it could have some emotional factors affecting them, too. But at the same time, the racers have a lot of muscle that needs a lot of oxygen. The higher metabolism that younger kids have [makes them] more prone to high-altitude sickness. The clients who stay in Vail or Aspen, they are much older, like forties, fifties, sixties. And they're not as athletic as the racers. They do not do any training. So their basic metabolism is low, so I believe they do not need as much oxygen.

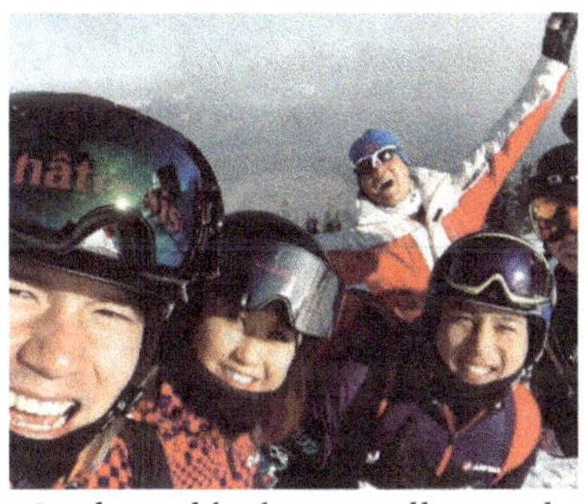

Smiles and high spirits all around.

Does anyone come from a high elevation in Japan, or is it mostly sea level?

Mostly sea level. Only some of them are from Nozawa. It's about 1,000 meters [3,281 feet], so it's much lower than Denver.

Is there a difference between the guests that come from Nozawa and the guests that come from sea level?

No. Whenever I see the doctor in the ER or the Copper clinic, they always say it's dehydration. No matter how much we tell them to keep hydrated, it's not enough.

What does the ER or clinic often give them besides fluids?

Oxygen. And they say it's okay to take over-the-counter headache medication.

How long are their visits to the hospital? Are they just a couple of hours, or do they stay overnight?

Just a couple of hours, or less than that.

Do they ski the next day?

Most of the time, the doctors say not to ski the next day. We carry a pulse oximeter in our office. We have twenty of them. We do not do this for the

Vail clients, because they don't get altitude sickness. We only do this for the guests staying in Summit County. When we [check them in], we distribute pulse oximeters, one per room. We encourage them to measure [their oxygen levels] every morning. Then, after the doctor's visit, the doctors say it's okay if your oxygen level is over 90% twenty minutes after getting off oxygen.

What's the lowest oxygen level you've seen on any of your skiers?

38. [He was] fifteen. He was at the ER. He was transferred to Denver by ambulance. He was there for about three nights, and he went back to Japan.

Was that the only time somebody had to go back to sea level?

Yes. But it sounds like he had a heart issue, which we didn't know [about].

What advice do you give to help them acclimate more effectively?

I encourage them to eat carbohydrates instead of getting a lot of oily foods. If you have a lot of French fries, it's very oily. It will take more time and blood to get to the stomach. So the blood flow doesn't go through the brain [well].

What about caffeine or other holistic remedies?

No. We have some repeat guests who had ... symptoms in past years, and we encourage them to visit a doctor in Japan [who] can prescribe ... Diamox. One of the ski coaches [from Japan] ... has to be here with his team. He has no choice. And he's [had] a lot of altitude sickness in the past. So we told him, "You should see a doctor and get Diamox prescribed, and start taking it before leaving Japan," and it's been working great.

Do your clients have any routines to prevent feeling this sickness?

Just check blood oxygen level every morning.

Do your regular clients acclimate more quickly each time?

They learn. We always see lower numbers of altitude sickness patients, because they learn what they need to do, like drinking a lot of water and checking their blood oxygen level. And only the numbers can tell. Even if they feel good, if the numbers are bad, if they go skiing, they will have a problem. Especially for the young kids. They [don't] trust what you say. As the years go by, the coaches will learn, and the kids will learn what they can and ... cannot do.

Is there anything different about the philosophy of treatment in Japan versus the United States?

You know what, we do not have altitude sickness in Japan. Only if you climb up Mt. Fuji in one day, it could happen, but not everyone does that. The highest elevation of one ski area in Japan is about 2,000 meters (6,600 feet). No one has experienced high-altitude sickness in Japan.

When I climbed Mt. Fuji, I saw a lot of people with cans of oxygen you can spray. Do you ever use or recommend that?

No. I don't think it works. If you breathe it for five minutes, it will work for five minutes. So I guess it's very effective if a ski racer uses it right before the start [of a race]. I believe some of our Vail clients [have seen] the bottle and have purchased it, but I've never heard anything about it, good or bad.

In closing, I asked Ryoko if she's noticed a change in her own physiology since living at high altitude, to which she replied that she is always impressed by her increased stamina and speed when she steps on a treadmill back at sea level. I asked her if she ever experiences symptoms upon coming back to high altitude from sea level. "No," she says, laughing. She doesn't typically engage in any strenuous activity the first day or two after traveling "because I'm lazy."

PART IX
BENEFITS OF ALTITUDE: AGING AND LONGEVITY

Beneficial Effects of Chronic Hypoxia

Living in Summit County, Colorado, has its perks: residents are within twenty to forty minutes of five world-class ski resorts, and some of the most beautiful Rocky Mountain trail systems are accessible right outside our back door. With endless opportunities for physical activity, it comes as no surprise that this is one of the healthiest communities in the country. This may also have something to do with the thin air.

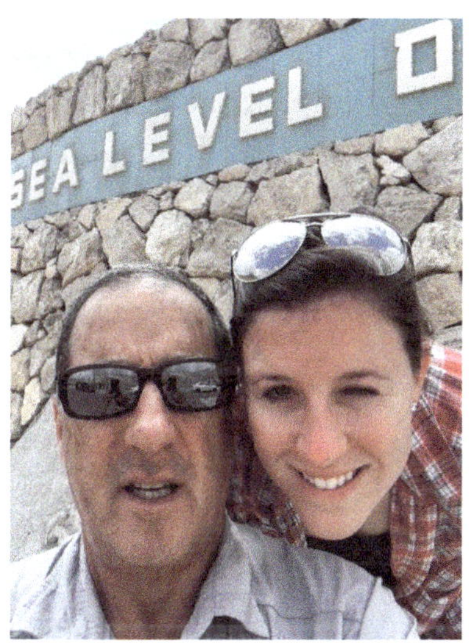

Dr. David Gray and daughter Dr. Kayla Van Der Kooi.

If you're a Summit County native, you have likely heard the terms **hypoxia** or **hypoxemia** mentioned a time or two. What do these mean? Simply put, these words describe the physiological condition that occurs when there is a deficiency of oxygen in the blood, resulting in decreased oxygen supply to the body's tissues.

While the acute effects of altitude can clearly have detrimental effects on one's physical wellbeing, there is emerging research demonstrating that chronic hypoxia may actually come with several health benefits. Longtime Summit County business owner and community pediatrician **Dr. Christine Ebert-Santos**, of Ebert Family Clinic in Frisco, has spent quite some time studying the effects of chronic high-altitude exposure. She recently attended and presented at the Chronic Hypoxia Symposium in La Paz, Bolivia, the highest capital city in the world.

First, it's important to understand the adaptations that occur in our bodies as a result of long-term hypoxia. The ability to maintain oxygen balance is essential to our survival, so how do those of us living in a place where each breath we take contains about a third fewer oxygen molecules survive?

Simply put, we beef up our ability to transport oxygen throughout our bodies. To do this, our kidneys, lungs, and brains increase their production of a hormone called erythropoietin, or EPO. This hormone signals the body to increase its production of red blood cells in the bone marrow. Red blood cells contain oxygen-binding hemoglobin proteins that deliver oxygen to the body's tissues. Thus, more red blood cells equal more oxygen-carrying capacity. In addition to increasing the ability to carry oxygen, our bodies also adapt on a cellular level by increasing the efficiency of energy-producing biochemical pathways and by decreasing the use of oxygen-consuming processes.[2] Furthermore, the response to chronic hypoxia stimulates the production of growth factors in the body that work to improve vascularization,[2] thus, increased ability for oxygenated blood to reach its destination.

So, what are the health benefits of this? To start, it appears that adaptation to continuous hypoxia has cardioprotective effects, conferring defense against lethal myocardial injury caused by acute ischemia (lack of blood flow) and the subsequent injury caused by return of blood to the affected area.[3] The exact mechanism of how this occurs is not well understood, but it seems that heart tissue adapts to be better able to tolerate episodes of ischemia, making it more resistant to damage that could otherwise be done by decreased blood flow that occurs during a heart attack. This same principle applied to ischemic brain damage when tested in rat subjects. Compared to their normoxic counterparts, rats pre-conditioned with hypoxia sustained less ischemic brain changes when subjected to carotid artery occlusion, suggesting neuroprotective effects of chronic hypoxia exposure.[4]

Additionally, it appears that altitude-adapted individuals may be better equipped to combat a pathological process known as endothelial dysfunction.[5] This process is a driving force in the development of atherosclerotic, coronary, and cerebrovascular artery disease. Altitude induces relative vasodilation of highlanders' blood vessels compared to lowlanders'.[2] A relaxing molecule known as nitric oxide, or NO, assists with causing this dilation, and in turn, the resultant dilated blood vessels produce more of this compound.[5] The molecule has protective effects on the inner linings of blood vessels and helps to decrease the production of pro-inflammatory cytokines that damage the endothelium.[5] This damage is what kickstarts the cascade that leads to atherosclerosis in our arteries. Thus, a constant state of hypoxia-induced vasodilation may in fact decrease one's risk of developing occlusive vascular disease.

A study of 2,789 men and 1,886 women, aged 14 to 85 years, showed a reduced risk of altitude sickness above age 46. The study controlled for age, sex, rate of ascent, final altitude, training status, and chemoreceptor responsiveness. 30 subjects were also evaluated again after a ten-year interval. Aging men showed a decreased response to hypoxia with less-pronounced desaturation. Men and women had a decreased cardiac response to low oxygen as they aged.[7]

The topics mentioned above highlight a few of the proposed mechanisms by which chronic hypoxia may be beneficial to our health. However, do keep in mind that there are potential detrimental effects, including an increased incidence of pulmonary hypertension as well as exacerbation of preexisting conditions such as COPD, structural heart defects, and sleep apnea, to name a few.[6] Research regarding the effects of chronic hypoxia on the human body is ongoing, and given its significance to those of us living at elevations of 9,000 feet (2,700 meters) and above, it is important to be aware of the impact our physical environments have on our health.

REFERENCES

1. Theodore, A. (2018). Oxygenation and mechanisms for hypoxemia. In G. Finlay (Ed.), UpToDate. Retrieved May 2, 2019, from https://www-uptodate-com.proxy.rvu.edu/contents/oxygenation-and-mechanisms-of-hypoxemia?search=hypoxia&source=search_ result&selectedTitle=1~150&usage_type=default&display_rank=1#H467959.

2. Michiels C. (2004). Physiological and pathological responses to hypoxia. The American journal of pathology, 164(6), 1875–1882. doi:10.1016/S0002-9440(10)63747-9. Retrieved May 2, 2019. https://www.ncbi.nlm.nih.gov/pmc/articles/PMC1615763.

3. Kolar, F. (2019). Molecular mechanism underlying the cardioprotective effects conferred by adaptation to chronic continuous and intermittent hypoxia. 7th Chronic Hypoxia Symposium Abstracts. pg 4. Retrieved May 2, 2019. http://zuniv.net/symposium7/Abstracts7CHS.pdf.

4. Das, K., Biradar, M. (2019). Unilateral common carotid artery occlusion and brain histopathology in rats pre-conditioned with sub chronic hypoxia. 7th Chronic Hypoxia Symposium Abstracts. pg 5. Retrieved May 2, 2019. http://zuniv.net/symposium7/Abstracts7CHS.pdf.

5. Gerstein, W. (2019). Endothelial dysfunction at high altitude. 7th Chronic Hypoxia Symposium Abstracts. pg 11. Retrieved May 7, 2019. http://zuniv.net/symposium7/Abstracts7CHS.pdf.

6. Hypoxemia. Cleveland Clinic. Updated March 7, 2018. Retrieved May 9, 2019. https://my.clevelandclinic.org/health/diseases/17727-hypoxemia.

7. Jean-Paul Richalet,1,2 and François J. Lhuissier, 1,2, High Altitude Medicine and biology June 2015.

From Mountains to Mars: Why High-Altitude Research Matters for Mars Missions

"THIN AIR"

You step out of your car at roughly 9,000 feet (2,700 meters) in Frisco, Colorado, and the first thing you notice isn't the mountain views, it's your breath. It comes faster, deeper, almost as if your body knows something you don't: the air pressure here is lower, and each breath delivers about 28% fewer oxygen molecules than at sea level.[1] This "thin air" triggers the same hypoxic (low-oxygen) stress that Mars settlers will face, where every habitat and spacesuit must carefully control both pressure and oxygen.[1,2,7,8] On Mars, the atmospheric pressure is less than 1% of that on Earth.

ACCLIMATIZATION

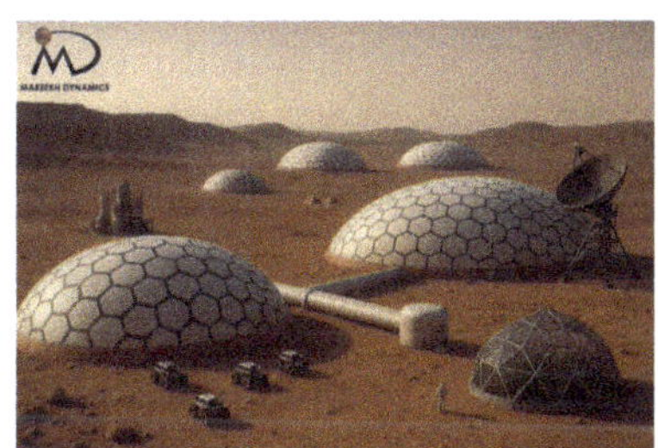

Craterhab base concept for housing on Mars.

On your first hike, your heart pounds harder than usual. That's your body's rapid response: breathing quickens, heart rate rises, and oxygen delivery ramps up to keep the entire body going.[1,2,4] Within twenty-four to forty-eight hours, your kidneys release erythropoietin (EPO), signaling the bone marrow to make more red blood cells.[1,3] This raises hemoglobin levels, enhancing oxygen transport. Over the following weeks, blood volume and hemoglobin continue to rise.[1,2,4] This is acclimatization, and it varies between individuals—an important consideration when selecting crew members for long-duration Mars missions.

SLEEP AND OXYGEN

At night, breathing becomes fragile. Many people develop "periodic breathing," or brief pauses that fragment sleep. Summit County residents often experience oxygen dips into the high 80s, lower than the approximately 90% seen in Denver and far below the typical 96%–98% at sea level.[1] These dips have real implications: hypoxia combined with sleep disruption can affect mood, stress, and cognitive performance, as seen in Antarctic "winter overs," where low oxygen and isolation have caused an up to 20% drop in certain cognitive task speeds and increased mood disturbances. Altitude sleep data is useful for researchers to determine extra nighttime buffers and habitat controls. Predicting and mitigating these person-specific patterns is key for astronaut safety and performance.[4,5]

FROM FRISCO TO THE FINAL FRONTIER

Frisco is not just known for its scenic views. This mountain town serves as a "living laboratory," allowing researchers to track oxygen saturation, breathing, heart rate, sleep, and exercise tolerance in residents and visitors. These insights can help engineers determine how much oxygen a Mars habitat should provide, and how quickly conditions can safely change after landing.[1,2,7,8] NASA spacecraft air pressures currently range from 8.2–4.7 psi, with oxygen comprising 21%–32% of that air, parameters informed in part by high-altitude research.[7,8] At the 7th Chronic Hypoxia Symposium in La Paz, Bolivia, at 12,000 feet (3,657 meters) elevation, the use of insights from high-altitude populations to enable the exploration of space was discussed. The sponsor and organizers were Drs. Gustavo Zubieta-Calleja and his daughter Natalia Zubieta De Urioste, who run the High Altitude Pulmonary & Pathology Institute there. Presenters and attendees came from sixteen countries and covered topics ranging from molecular biology to genetics.

A presentation on "BioSpace-Forming" identified chronic hypoxia as a "fundamental tool" that "gives humans and other species an advantage on earth and beyond." Dr. Zubieta explained that the space station is engineered to have the barometric pressure (760 mmHg) and oxygen content of sea level. When the astronauts change into their spacesuits to work outside the ship, they experience a pressure drop of over 200 mmHg in the laborious process of donning the suit. Seeing that millions of inhabitants are healthy at 486 mmHg in Bolivia, Dr. Zubieta asserts that maintaining lower pressures and lower oxygen levels in the space station would be economical and promote the health of the astronauts. Several altitude scientists see this as a future that "uncouples biology and physics."

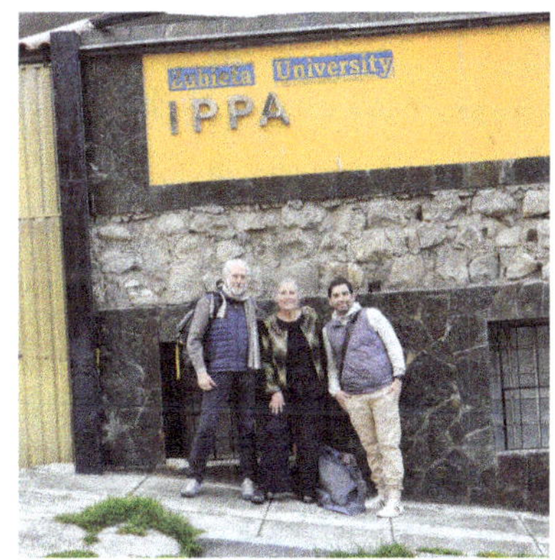

Dr. Christine Ebert-Santos, in front of the High Altitude Pulmonary & Pathology Institute in La Paz, Bolivia, with Michele Samaja, PhD, from the University of Milan and Cristian Arias Reyes, PhD, from the Seattle Children's Research Institute, presenting their research at the 9th Chronic Hypoxia Symposium & 1st High-Altitude Space Physiology Symposia in February 2025.

MODELING MARS CONDITIONS

Researchers combine data from high-altitude locations, Antarctic stations, and Mars analog habitats, like HI-SEAS in Hawaii, to build predictive models. These models provide guidelines for when oxygen supplementation or workload adjustments are needed to optimize safety while completing tasks.[4–6,9] They also help develop "operations playbooks" for simulating life on Mars,[10] set habitat air pressure and oxygen guidelines,[7,8] define spacesuit safety limits,[4,6,11] and better understand how the human body responds to spaceflight and space living.[2,5,9,12,13] For example, extravehicular activity (EVA) suits—spacesuits used for work outside the spacecraft—typically operate at about 4.3 psi with 100% oxygen. While this allows astronauts to breathe in low-pressure environments, prolonged use can lead to overheating, dehydration, and higher risk of injuries.[11]

The gravitational pull on Mars is 38% of that on Earth. Solar radiation, and the more dangerous Galactic Cosmic Radiation of alpha particles from distant supernovae, are hundreds of times greater than on Earth due to Mars's lack of a magnetic field or protective atmosphere. A breeze on Mars could barely move a blade of grass. Global dust storms occur every few years and last months, devastating the surface.

At the 9th Chronic Hypoxia Symposium & 1st High-Altitude Space Physiology Symposia in La Paz in 2025, Dr. Akbar Hussain presented his Craterhab design for accommodations in austere high-altitude environments and eventually on Mars.

Before embarking on the long journey to distant space, astronauts could be acclimatized in facilities located at 5,000 meters (16,400 feet) near mines in the Andes.

LIMITATIONS

Most high-altitude studies are conducted over weeks or months, while Mars missions could last years and require hundreds of participants to collectively have the skills to be self-sustaining. Due to planetary rotations, travel to Mars is only feasible once every twenty-six months. Messages from Mars take seven to forty-five minutes to arrive on Earth. Individual differences in acclimatization, long-term cognitive effects, and combined stressors like radiation or microgravity are not fully captured. Longer-duration studies at high altitudes, combined with simulated Martian habitats and spacesuit trials, are needed to refine safety parameters.

CONCLUSION

High-altitude research gives scientists a window into human maladaptive and adaptive responses to low-oxygen, low-pressure conditions on Earth, and is directly relevant to anticipating health risks and necessary countermeasures for human habitation on Mars.

REFERENCES

1. Ebert-Santos C. High-Altitude Pulmonary Edema in Mountain Community Residents. High Alt Med Biol. 2017 Sep;18(3):278-284. doi: 10.1089/ham.2016.0100. Epub 2017 Aug 28. PMID: 28846035.

2. Le Roy B, Martin-Krumm C, Pinol N, Dutheil F, Trousselard M. Human challenges to adaptation to extreme professional environments: A systematic review. Neurosci Biobehav Rev. 2023;146:105054. doi:10.1016/j.neubiorev.2023.105054.

3. Roach RC, Hackett PH. Frontiers of hypoxia research: acute mountain sickness. J Exp Biol. 2001 Sep;204(Pt 18):3161-70. doi: 10.1242/jeb.204.18.3161. PMID: 11581330.

4. Mairesse O, MacDonald-Nethercott E, Neu D et al. Preparing for Mars: Human sleep and performance during a 13-month stay in Antarctica. Sleep. 2019;42(1). doi:10.1093/sleep/zsy206.

5. Pagel JI, Choukèr A. Effects of isolation and confinement on humans—Implications for manned space explorations. J Appl Physiol (1985). 2016;120(12):1449-1457. doi:10.1152/japplphysiol.00928.2015.

6. Dunn Rosenberg J, Jannasch A, Binsted K, Landry S. Biobehavioral and psychosocial stress changes during three 8–12 month spaceflight analog missions with Mars-like conditions of isolation and confinement. Front Physiol. 2022;13:898841. doi:10.3389/fphys.2022.898841.

7. Waligora JM, Horrigan DJ, Nicogossian A. The physiology of spacecraft and space suit atmosphere selection. Acta Astronaut. 1991;23:171-177. doi:10.1016/0094-5765(91)90116-M.

8. Morgenthaler GW, Fester DA, Cooley CG. An assessment of habitat pressure, oxygen fraction, and EVA suit design for space operations. Acta Astronaut. 1994;32(1):39-49. doi:10.1016/0094-5765(94)90146-5.

9. Sarma MS, Shelhamer M. The human biology of spaceflight. Am J Hum Biol. 2024;36(3):e24048. doi:10.1002/ajhb.24048.

10. Lim DSS, Abercromby AFJ, Kobs Nawotniak SE et al. The BASALT research program: Designing and developing mission elements in support of human scientific exploration of Mars. Astrobiology. 2019;19(3):245-259. doi:10.1089/ast.2018.1869.

11. Stirling L, Arezes P, Anderson A. Implications of space suit injury risk for developing computational performance models. Aerosp Med Hum Perform. 2019;90(6):553-565. doi:10.3357/AMHP.5221.2019.

12. Cassaro A, Pacelli C, Aureli L et al. Antarctica as a reservoir of planetary analogue environments. Extremophiles. 2021;25(5-6):437-458. doi:10.1007/s00792-021-01245-w.

13. Fairén AG, Davila AF, Lim D et al. Astrobiology through the ages of Mars: The study of terrestrial analogues to understand the habitability of Mars. Astrobiology. 2010;10(8):821-843. doi:10.1089/ast.2009.0440.

14. Akbar Hussain M, Ayaz Hussain M, Mehdi Hussain M, Fatima R, Carretero R, eds. Craterhab Technology: Adapting Martian Habitat Systems to Combat Chronic Hypoxia in High-Altitude Mining in the Andes - A White Paper. Mareekh Dynamics. Published June 3, 2024. Accessed August 15, 2025. https://www.mareekh.com/post/craterhab-technology-adapting-martian-habitat-systems-to-combat-chronic-hypoxia-in-high-altitude-mi.

Contributing Authors

Atkinson, Catherine, PA-C. *How Do You Define a Good Night's Sleep?: An Introduction to the SleepImage Ring (Interview with Dr. Neale Lange)*

Axmann Grabinger, Angi, NP. *High-Altitude Cerebral Edema (HACE) and Metabolism at Altitude: Can Nutrition Help?*

Bergin, Amanda, FNP. *HAST: The High-Altitude Simulation Test*

Bice, Claire, PA-C. *A Survival Guide for Driving the I-70 Corridor*

Bradfield, Jenna, PA-C. *How Altitude Can Permanently Change Your Brain*

Gordon, Sarah, PA-C. *Altitude as Asthma Treatment*

Kligerman, Taylor, PA-C. *Can I Ever Go Back Up to High Altitude Again? Recurrence Risk of HAPE and HARPE*

Luger, Autumn, PA-C. *Doc Talk: The Art of Saving Vacations*

Miller, Joel, PA-C. *Pre-acclimatization: A Synopsis of Dr. Peter Hackett's Lecture at the Wilderness Medical Society*

Pawar, Noor, PA-C. *"Eructile" Dysfunction at Altitude: Low Barometric Pressures Worsen Discomfort for Those Who Can't Burp*

Schara, Delaney, PA-C. *Closer to the Sun: The Dermatological Benefits and Consequences of Living at High Altitude*

Slaton, Lyrin, PA-C. *From Mountains to Mars: Why High-Altitude Research Matters for Mars Missions*

Smeele, Rianne, BSN, RN. *Can I Take My Child up a Fourteener?*

Transue, Laundon, PA-C. *Watch Out for Flying Discs: How High Altitude Changes Flight*

Van Der Kooi, Kayla, MD. *Beneficial Effects of Chronic Hypoxia*

Van Steyn, Laura, PA-C. *Mountain Kids Are Smaller*

Zak, Courtney, PA-C. *Dogs and the High-Country Winter*